CONDOM

Paul Allen is a freelance writer and author. His work has appeared in *The Times*, *The Guardian* and *New Internationalist*, among other publications. In 2007, he wrote *Your Ethical Business: How to Plan, Start and Succeed in a Company with a Conscience* (ngo.media). He currently lives in East London, where he writes about social, ethical and environmental issues for the national and international press.

NEW INTERNATIONALIST

Trigger Issues
One small item – one giant impact

Other titles in the series:

Diamonds

Football

Kalashnikov

Mosquito

T-shirt

About the New Internationalist

The **New Internationalist** is an independent not-for-profit publishing co-operative. Our mission is to report on issues of global justice. We publish informative current affairs and popular reference titles, complemented by world food, photography and gift books as well as calendars, diaries, maps and posters – all with a global justice world view.

If you like this **Trigger Issue** book you'll also love the **New Internationalist** magazine. Each month it takes a different subject such as Trade Justice, Nuclear Power or Iraq, exploring and explaining the issues in a concise way; the magazine is full of photos, charts and graphs as well as music, film and book reviews, country profiles, interviews and news.

To find out more about the **New Internationalist**, visit our website at: **www.newint.org**

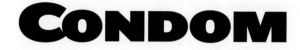

CONDOM

Paul Allen

NEW INTERNATIONALIST

Trigger Issues: Condom
First published in the UK in 2007 by
New Internationalist™ Publications Ltd
Oxford OX4 1BW, UK
www.newint.org
New Internationalist is a registered trade mark.

Series editor: Troth Wells
Design by New Internationalist Publications Ltd.

Printed on recycled paper by TJ International, UK
who hold environmental accreditation ISO 14001.

British Library Cataloguing-in-Publication Data.
A catalogue record for this book is available from the British Library.

Library of Congress Cataloguing-in-Publication Data.
A catalogue for this book is available from the Library of Congress.

ISBN: 978-1-904456-76-6

Contents

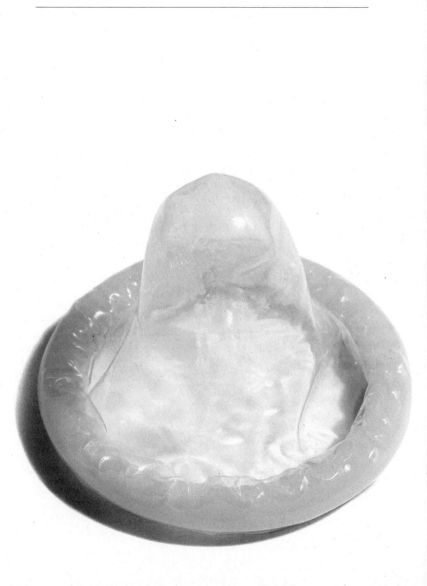

1

The birth of birth control

When Christopher Columbus returned to Europe from the New World at the turn of the 16th century, his crew was carrying more than just plundered gold and slaves. Western explorers had long been infecting indigenous populations with foreign viruses. But this time around, it was the local people who unwittingly passed on a lethal infection. As his men climbed ashore in Spain, Columbus's deadly cargo was unleashed: syphilis. With ferocious speed, the disease swept across Europe. Spread by sexual intercourse, its victims suffered a slow and painful death. In the absence of any effective treatment, the sores could worsen so dramatically that victims of later-stage syphilis were often mistakenly presumed to have leprosy. For centuries, a common treatment was mercury, which had the unfortunate side-effect of death by poisoning.

For the medical profession, this virulent disease presented an urgent challenge. With sexual intercourse increasingly resembling a game of Russian roulette, the race began to find a cure. In 1564, Gabriele Fallopio (who gives his name to fallopian tubes) instead proposed a preventive. In a work published in 1564, two years after his death, the Italian anatomist described a linen sheath to ward off venereal disease.

While Fallopio provides the first written record of condoms in European history, it is very likely that they have been with us for much longer. A crude cave drawing at Les Combarelles, France, shows an apparently sheathed man dating from between 15,000 BCE and 10,000 BCE. In ancient Egypt, a device resembling a condom may have been used as far back as the XIX Dynasty (1350-1200 BCE). The Egyptians may even have dyed them different colors.

We will probably never know exactly what the ancient civilizations *did* with these sheaths, however. Some may have been simply penis protectors, which have been used since prehistoric times to protect the wearer during combat, as well as against insect bites or evil spirits. They may also have served purely decorative purposes or acted as lucky charms. Even today, some Dani people in West Papua wear nothing but a *koteka* – a long, upward-pointing penis sheath made of gourd.

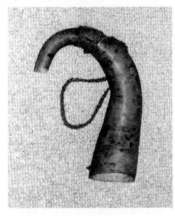

Koteka – penis sheath.

Nevertheless, while disease prevention is a relatively modern use for condoms, the need for birth control has been with us since time immemorial. This desire to limit family size, due to various physical, emotional, social or economic reasons, suggests that civilizations would have been experimenting with contraception long before Fallopio's linen creations. Along with more natural approaches, such as the rhythm method, *coitus interruptus* (withdrawal followed by ejaculation) and vaginal douching, it is possible that early peoples also experimented with other more artificial ways to block insemination.

Most evidence, however, shows that these early efforts were focused on women's anatomy. Women in ancient South American civilizations, for example, fashioned themselves a female contraceptive made out of a cut-off seedpod. Upper-class women in ancient Egypt are said to have used crocodile-dung pessaries and irrigated the vagina with honey and sodium bicarbonate. Another kind of pessary, popular in African pre-industrial societies, was a solid object to block the cervix; women also made plugs of chopped grass or cloth. In Japan, prostitutes are said to have used balls of bamboo tissue-paper, while wool was preferred by Muslim and Greek women. These techniques evidently enjoyed some success. Until the development of the diaphragm, the sea sponge – which was wrapped in silk with a string attached – used by ancient Jews was considered one of the most effective contraceptives in use.

This emphasis on female protection continued for several centuries. In the Middle Ages, magicians are said to have advised women to wear the testicles of a weasel on their thighs or hang its amputated foot from around their necks. Other 'lucky' charms included ground cat-liver, flax lint tied in a cloth and soaked in menstrual blood, and the anus of a hare. It was also believed that a woman could avoid pregnancy by walking three times around the spot where a pregnant wolf had urinated. As recently as the 1800s, some women in Canada would brew dried beaver testicle in alcohol to create a contraceptive potion.

While many of these rituals appear absurd today, some had a genuinely scientific basis. When researchers discovered women in a particular Mexican tribe were apparently avoiding conception by eating a certain wild yam, for example, they studied the vegetable further. The hormone present in these yams, with the addition of estrogen, subsequently led to the first birth control pill. In China, some women drank lead and mercury to control fertility, but this often resulted in sterility or death.

The earliest surviving oral account of *male* contraception appears rather less grounded in reality. According to legend, when he wasn't busy getting Hercules to kill the Minotaur, King Minos of Crete was said to have a rather embarrassing personal problem. Whenever he had sex, the king would ejaculate snakes and scorpions in his seed which killed all his lovers. His personal physician therefore invented a receptacle made from a goat's bladder which would catch his sperm, and thereby protect his lover.

Life-savers

As syphilis raged through 16th-century Europe, contraception was for the first time not simply a matter of preventing new life, but also of avoiding death. In Fallopio's groundbreaking work *De Morbo Gallico* (literally 'On the French disease', the Italian slang for syphilis) he described a small linen sheath, which fitted either over the glans of the penis or (more painfully) was inserted into the urethra. He claimed to have trialed it on 1,100 men and none was infected with syphilis. In 1597, medical scholar Hercules Saxonia improved on Fallopio's primitive designs by introducing the first spermicide. He advised soaking the linen sheaths in a chemical solution and allowing them to dry before use.

During the second half of the 17th century, linen began to be replaced by stretched animal gut. Sheep, lamb, calf and goat intestine were a readily available waste product from the slaughterhouse. They also felt much more like a 'second skin', although they were looser and had to be tied with a ribbon. At the same time, there were also

'To quench the heat of Venus's fire, and yet preserve the flame of love's desire.'

Anon.

LIFE THROUGH A LENS

The 17th century welcomed another important medical discovery. While early condoms were most likely being used for disease prevention *and* birth control, contemporary scientists actually knew very little about the mechanics of conception, ie the fertilization of an egg by a sperm. In 1677, a discovery by Antonie van Leeuwenhoek advanced scientific thinking – and kick-started a controversy in the history of condoms. Using a primitive microscope, the Dutch scientist was the first person to find *animalcula*, or spermatozoa. In *Looking for Doctor Condom*, W E Kruck suggests 'the cause-and-effect relationship between intercourse and conception was (previously) well-known but not understood'. With van Leeuwenhoek's discovery of sperm, the link between condoms and birth control was officially sealed. Among many religious thinkers, the implications of a man's seed 'dying' in condoms still provokes outrage to this day. ◆

experimentations with fish bladders.

The early condoms were not easy to make. After being soaked, inverted, softened, scraped and inflating, the stomach lining then had to be dried and cut into shape. It was an expensive process, and though reusable, they were costly. Very few men would have been able to have them tailor-made from scratch.

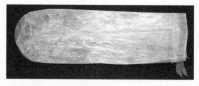

Early condom made of gut
and tied with ribbon.

Nevertheless, they were effective. And beyond this efficacy at disease prevention, it's clear that condoms were also recognized as a means of birth control. A 17th-century poem by the son of an English bishop praised the liberating effect that condoms would have on young women, freed from the 'big Belly, and the squawking brat'. But the new contraceptive was also highly advantageous for men, regardless of wealth or class. Poor men were eager to escape the financial drain of additional mouths to feed. Besides the question of heirs, wealthier gentlemen were concerned not to damage their reputation in society with children from illicit sexual liaisons.

Casanova's condoms

The renowned 18th-century lover Giacomo Casanova was certainly well experienced with condoms. Although he hated them at first – dubbing them *redingotes Anglaises* ('English riding coats') and cursing their smell and inconvenience – he changed his mind later in life.

In 1758, he praised their effectiveness in freeing him

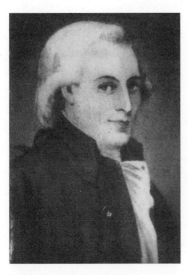

from any more heirs or venereal disease. 'Ten years ago, I would have called this an invention of the devil, but now I believe that its inventor must have been a good man,' he wrote in his diaries. The Italian lothario wasn't beyond trying other methods of contraception, however. Perhaps most famously, he experimented with using half a lemon as a cervical cap.

This was surprisingly effective, and has since been proven to be scientifically sound. In 2002, Australian scientist Roger Short even suggested that lemon juice could be an effective and cheap microbicide to help reduce the spread of HIV/AIDS in the developing world. In studies, he reported that a solution of 10-per-cent lemon juice produced a 1,000-fold reduction in HIV activity in a lab sample. He claimed that half a teaspoon of the highly acidic juice wiped out two teaspoons of sperm in just 30 seconds.

THE REAL DOCTOR CONDOM?

No one knows where the word 'condom' originated. However, one popular – if unsubstantiated – theory is the existence of a certain 'Dr Condom'.

According to different sources, he was either the physician to King Charles II, a colonel during his reign – or both. Author Jeannette Parisot concluded that the inventor of the first sheep-gut sheath was Colonel Quondom, a Royalist army physician.

Quondom reputedly survived the English Civil War, but to avoid being identified with the Royalist defeat, he retired from the army and changed his name to Dr Cundum.

As a physician, he had allegedly created the membranous sheath to provide the King with a means of preventing more illegitimate offspring. Given the prevalence of syphilis, however, they may also have been to prevent sexually transmitted infection.

Historically at least, this theory tallies approximately with the discovery at Dudley Castle of the world's oldest surviving

The early condom trade

By the early 18th century, London had become the center of a thriving international condom trade. Its captains of industry were a certain Mrs Perkins and Mrs Phillips, two bitter rivals who sold to apothecaries, ambassadors and travelers, and claimed to have received large orders from 'France, Spain, Portugal, Italy and other foreign places'.

condom fragments, dating to 1640. A more complete condom found in Sweden, dating from the same year, is on display at the Tyrolean County Museum in Austria.

There are many other theories to explain the word 'condom'. One is that when Catherine de Medici married Henry II of France, she brought her minister Gondi and the architect Bernardo Buontalenti. Together, they are purported to have started producing waxed protections to be used as condoms, which the French began to call 'gondons'.

Other theories trace the word condom from the Latin verb 'condere' (to contain) or 'condos' (receptacle). Some people believe they are simply named after the French town, Condom. Others cite the Persian 'Kendu' or 'Kondu', meaning a long storage vessel made from animal intestine, as the original etymology. In 1972, even *Playboy* magazine contributed a theory, suggesting the word comes from 'conundrum': a riddle, difficult to put on. ◆

For poorer customers, there was 'Miss Jenny' who sold washed second-hand condoms.

To guard yourself from shame or fear,
Votaries to Venus, fasten here;
None in our wares e'er found a flaw,
Self-preservation's nature's law.

A common 18th-century advertising slogan.

In his *History of the Condom*, Dr H Youssef writes that the sheath was widely praised in erotic poetry of the period, and often referred to as 'the preservative machine' or simply 'armour'. Among its adherents was James Boswell, the famous biographer of English literary giant Samuel Johnson. On 10 May 1763, the fast-living Boswell recounts how he picked up a strong, young, jolly damsel, led her to Westminster Bridge and there 'in armour, complete did I enjoy her upon this noble edifice'.

Getting a grip

By the mid-19th century, the European scramble for colonies was in full swing. Among the indigenous goods plundered and brought back by the colonial powers was rubber, which was originally from South America.

As a base material, rubber is extremely sticky and difficult to handle. But in 1839, Charles Goodyear, the man whose name is now synonymous with car tires, experimentally dropped a mixture of rubber and sulfur onto a hot stove. What he discovered was that the resulting mass was a very strong, stable and elastic material. The discovery of this process, known as vulcanization, revolutionized condom production almost overnight. Unlike meticulously handcrafted animal-gut sheaths, vulcanized rubber was not simply quick to make, but it could also be stretched and produced much more cheaply.

Nevertheless, the earliest 'rubber johnnies' were still very different to our modern condom. To start, these creations had the thickness of bicycle inner tubes and seams down the sides. In *Johnny Come Lately*, French writer Jeanette Parisot describes two different versions. The first 'consists of a delicate membranous tube which corresponds to the dimensions of the erect penis, is sealed at the front end and at the rear end usually has a fastening device (ribbons)'. The second was a successor to Fallopio's 'tip' condom: 'When filled with water, the condom has the shape, either of an egg from which a small section has been cut, or the glans penis. When the condom is in use (a) ring fits so tightly around the glans that the condom cannot slip off during intercourse.'

The inherent problem with 'tip' condoms was the need to have them tailor-made. This involved a trip to the doctor to have the penis measured, and then the rigmarole of ensuring you bought exactly the right size. They also did not provide the same amount of protection against venereal disease as a full-length condom.

In the early days, rubber condoms were still beyond

KING OF CONDOMS

In 1865, Julius Schmid, a poor German-Jewish immigrant, arrived in the United States. He was 17 years old. After finding work at a sausage-maker's in New York, the young entrepreneur began to make and sell 'skins', condoms made from animal guts – a European phenomenon which had yet to reach the US. He then pioneered a new kind of safe, vulcanized rubber sheath, which gradually grew in popularity. By 1918, when condoms were legalized in America for disease prevention (but not contraception), Schmid was selling condoms to European troops. In World War II, the US Government made Schmid official condom supplier to the US armed forces. Soon, his business was earning $900,000 a year (equivalent to $11 million, or £5.7 million, in today's currency). The impoverished immigrant had become a multi-millionaire. In 1955, Schmid, then 73, handed over the reins of the company to his two sons, Carl and Julius Junior. ◆

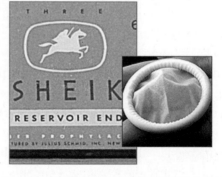

Schmid condom.

the means of most everyday men. Partly because of this, *coitus interruptus* was one of the most common methods of contraception in the world at this time, even though it is by no means effective. But as advances in manufacturing speeded up and costs came down, so the condom gradually captured the public imagination. By the turn of the century, new innovations were also improving the manufacturing process. In 1901, the year of Queen Victoria's death, the first teat-ended condoms (designed to hold ejaculate) were made by dipping glass moulds into a liquid rubber solution.

HOW IT WORKS

Today's latex condoms are disposable, easy to use and highly effective – so long as they are used correctly. The World Health Organization gives the following advice for wearers:

◆ Make sure that the condom is of good quality and not past its expiry date.

◆ Open the packet carefully so the condom does not tear.

◆ Squeeze the tip of the condom before unrolling it on to the erect penis.

◆ After ejaculation, hold the rim of the condom and pull the penis out while still hard.

◆ Do not use oil-based lubricants (stick to water-based, such as K-Y Jelly).

CONDOM • TRIGGER ISSUES

Latex love

Arguably the biggest revolution in condom manufacturing history was really just a clever shortcut. By the early 20th century, condoms were becoming more popular but they were still rather cumbersome and expensive. Thanks to Goodyear's invention, these were now made by turning sticky rubber sap (properly known as latex) into vulcanized rubber. But in the 1930s, scientists developed a way to skip this process – and turn the liquid latex straight into condoms.

No one knows exactly who pioneered the first latex condom, but the results were superlative. Latex proved better than rubber in every possible way. Not only was it cheaper, lighter, and more durable, it was also more

---

IN THE TRASH

Latex and sperm are both biodegradable, but condoms contain added ingredients, such as lubricants and stabilizers, which mean they need to be disposed of carefully. HIV/AIDS charity Avert recommends that condoms should be wrapped in tissue or toilet paper and put with the trash. Condoms should not be flushed down the toilet as they may cause blockages in the sewage system and also damage marine life. Condoms made from polyurethane, a plastic material, are not biodegradable at all. ◆

---

enjoyable to wear and easier to make. Indeed, the simplicity of making latex condoms rapidly led to much greater automation in production. Conveyor belts of glass moulds were simply dipped into liquid latex and dried before going into hot air chambers for vulcanization. As output surged, so prices plummeted. The resulting condoms were tougher and thinner, simultaneously offering the wearer even more sensation and greater protection.

In 1949, a Japanese firm introduced the first colored condom. The following year, the first lubricated condom was launched in the UK by Durex. In 1973, the first textured condoms were introduced to the market. Continual innovations since then mean that today, we have more choice than ever.

While latex remains the material of choice for most condoms worldwide, there are now innumerable variations in color, flavor, size, thickness and texture. For people allergic to latex, there are even polyurethane condoms, although these have a greater risk of breaking or slipping. One solution is 'double-bagging' – wearing an animal gut condom (still available from specialist stores) beneath a regular latex condom.

So, there were plenty of condoms and plenty of choice, but how to get people to use them?

2 Rubber revolution

Before the 20th century, condom manufacture was labor-intensive, expensive and therefore only wealthy men tended to use the prophylactics. By the early 1900s, technological advances had made condoms cheaper, more available and easier to use. They were also reusable and increasingly effective at disease prevention and birth control. A much bigger hurdle to overcome, however, was their social stigma. For centuries, condoms had been synonymous with male promiscuity. Designed to stop licentious men catching diseases from prostitutes or creating unwanted pregnancies, they were hardly considered a proper choice for a morally upstanding gentleman. For many people, the idea of using a condom was simply out of the question.

Across the sexual divide, however, different ideas were forming. By the early 1900s, the birth control movement had begun to gain momentum among women in the UK. In

MARVELOUS MARIE?

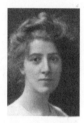

Marie Stopes is one of the most influential figures in the history of birth control. Born in Edinburgh, Scotland, in 1880, she studied palaeo-botany before turning her attention to family planning. While still unmarried, she published *Married Love* in 1918, a guide to a happy and enjoyable sexual life. Her driving philosophy was freedom, sexual satisfaction and enjoyable motherhood for all women. This led her to open the UK's first family planning clinic, the Mothers' Clinic, in north London in 1921.

The clinic offered a free advice service to married women and also gathered scientific data about contraception. It also marked the start of a new era in which couples, for the first time, could reliably take control of their fertility. At the time, Stopes received a frosty reception from many in the male-dominated medical profession (one described her works as 'practical handbooks of prostitution'), but she persevered tirelessly, writing further books on contraception, founding the Society for Constructive Birth Control and even chaining a copy

1921 Marie Stopes (see box 'Marvelous Marie?') opened the first birth control clinic in London with the slogan 'children by choice, not chance', and by the outbreak of World War Two, there were 69 family planning clinics across the country.

of her book *Roman Catholic Methods of Birth Control* to the front of Westminster Cathedral.

She also befriended Margaret Sanger (see p 52), a fellow birth-control activist who had been chased out of her native US on obscenity charges. While Stopes is recognized as one of the pioneers of women's free choice over birth control, she was less liberal in her views on who should be allowed to procreate. A strong advocate of eugenics, she believed that those 'unfit for parenthood' should be sterilized and added that she would 'legislate compulsory sterilization of the insane, feeble-minded... revolutionaries... half-castes'. She even opposed her son's marriage because his wife had a minor eye condition.

Supporters argue that her views on eugenics need to be understood within their historic context, namely before Nazi Germany's eugenics program was practiced on Jews, gypsies, homosexuals and mentally and physically disabled people. ◆

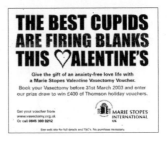

The expansion of birth control centers led to a much-needed, more open dialogue about sex and reproduction. Nevertheless, a major obstacle to contraception was that men were simply unused (and therefore unwilling) to take responsibility for their sexual urges. The very idea of a man having to quell his passions to put on a condom was still very far from the norm. For a whole generation of young men, however, all that was about to change.

Condoms in the wars

By the outbreak of World War One, the efficacy of condoms in disease prevention was well known. For military commanders, worried about keeping soldiers out on the battlefield, this was a very big tick in their favor.

In 1917, at a meeting of the Imperial War Conference, Allied military leaders acknowledged that venereal diseases were seriously impeding the fighting capacity of the forces. In that year alone, 23,000 British soldiers were hospitalized for treatment. The French Government had reported over a million cases of syphilis or gonorrhea since the start of the War. As a result, the European forces immediately began supplying condoms to the men.

In America, the question of condom distribution provoked a heated debate. In the end, the secretary of the navy, Josephus Daniels, rejected the idea – fearing that it would corrupt the troops' morals. Instead, they were to be encouraged to abstain. As an extra incentive to 'behave', American soldiers were told they would be court-martialed if they contracted a venereal disease. Nevertheless, in *No Magic Bullet*, historian and author Allan M Brandt reports that 383,000 US soldiers were diagnosed with venereal diseases between April 1917 and December 1919 and the US forces lost seven million days of active duty.

The moral tide was turning even in America, however. And while Daniels was on vacation, his then undersecretary (and future president), Franklin Roosevelt, authorized chemical prophylactics for sailors. Although well intentioned, these proved largely useless.

By World War Two, the US had learned its lesson. With the slogan 'Put it on before you put it in', servicemen were actively encouraged to use condoms. British soldiers had already found another meaning to this motto; by placing a condom over a gun's barrel, they could keep the weapon dry and prevent it from corroding or icing up. Condoms were issued to soldiers during the D-Day landings in 1944 for that very reason.

A serious problem with the policy of condom promotion

was a shortage of rubber, which threatened to halt the supply to the troops. But despite fears that the rubber would literally be stretched too thin (and predictable calls from the Roman Catholic Church for their withdrawal), the condoms kept on coming.

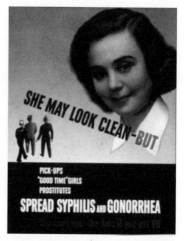

There are various unsubstantiated rumors about condom use during wartime. One story goes that Soviet leader Josef Stalin asked British Prime Minister Winston Churchill to help alleviate the condom shortage in the Russian army. Churchill allegedly agreed, ordering a British manufacturer to have a special batch made twice as large as normal. These were to be clearly labeled 'Made in Britain' and 'Size: Medium'.

In Nazi Germany, meanwhile, where Aryan mothers were being actively encouraged to produce more offspring for the new Reich, contraception was strictly *verboten*. Nevertheless, while a decree from SS commander Heinrich Himmler directly forbade the sale of condoms

> 'Only sailors wear condoms, baby.'
>
> *Austin Powers, International Man of Mystery.*

in public places, an exception was made for members of the army. At the same time, the authorities in France were also concerned about low birth rates, and banned abortion and all contraception.

The war years saw a boom in condom use, but this did nothing to change the condom's image as a tool of sexual dalliance; the transition to domestic life was still a long way off. This was delayed even further thanks to another revolutionary discovery. In 1929, Dr Alexander Fleming isolated what became known as the antibiotic penicillin from a fungal mould. By 1940, the Scotsman's 'magic bullet' was ready for commercial use. As well as revolutionizing modern medical practice, the antibiotic had a seismic impact on the popularity of the condom. For the first time, there was an effective medical treatment for syphilis, gonorrhea and a whole host of other STDs (sexually transmitted diseases – now referred to as STIs – 'infections'). Thanks to penicillin, sexual health in the UK improved dramatically in the 1940s and 1950s. For many, however, condoms seemed increasingly redundant.

The sexual revolution

After the economic hardships and sober reflection of the post-war years, the 1960s was a time of fresh optimism for a generation in the Western world. Shaking off the horrors of the past, young people were increasingly embracing the concept of freedom through various channels, such as drugs, music and sex. Indeed, this era is often dubbed the 'sexual revolution'. Historian David Allyn describes the relaxation in sexual morality as a time of 'coming-out' about premarital sex, masturbation, erotic fantasies, pornography use and homosexuality.

While the scale of this 'revolution' has been most certainly exaggerated over time, there is no doubt that new attitudes to sex were emerging in affluent Western societies. Within this movement, one of the most influential developments was the arrival of the oral contraceptive pill (see p 84), which for the first time put a reliable and convenient method of birth control into women's hands.

Sexual intercourse began
In nineteen sixty-three
(which was rather late for me) –
Between the end of the Chatterley ban
And the Beatles' first LP.

Philip Larkin, *Annus Mirabilis.*

For the condom, the arrival of the pill was yet another blow. The combination of laissez-faire attitudes to sex, an effective contraceptive tablet and better antibiotics sidelined the rubber sheath even further. Despite side-effects for some users, the pill was convenient to take, didn't detract from sexual pleasure and of course did not require the man to do anything at all. As a result, in the decade when Austin Powers would have been at his most 'shagadelic', sales of condoms actually plummeted.

This decline in popularity continued for almost two decades. But condoms were by no means finished. Nearly 500 years after one lethal disease had brought about their creation, another killer was about to put them firmly back on the map.

HIV/AIDS

No-one knows for sure where the Human Immuno-deficiency Virus (HIV) originated. What is understood is that, in 1978, a number of gay men in the US and Sweden, and heterosexual men in Tanzania and Haiti, all began developing rare infections and cancers which seemed resistant to any treatment. By the early 1980s, the death toll was rising fast. Initially, doctors were stumped. Linking the outbreak to its earliest occurrence in gay men, the condition was initially dubbed GRID (gay-related immune deficiency) or simply 'gay cancer'.

In fact, scientists had already unwittingly isolated the earliest case of AIDS. It had been found in a patient in Kinshasa, in what is now the Democratic Republic of Congo, in 1959. This discovery suggested that the multitude of global HIV infections all shared a common origin in Africa. That primary source, however, was not human. In 1999, scientists reported that chimpanzees were the origin of the HIV-1 virus, and that it had at some point crossed species from chimps to humans. The most commonly accepted theory is that the virus was transferred to hunters when they killed and ate the animals, either by blood getting into cuts or wounds on the hunter.

Faced with an incurable and deadly disease, scare stories abounded. Fueled by hysterical reports in the media, many people believed the virus could be caught from the most unlikely sources: toilet seats, gay plumbers 'infecting' a cistern or even communion wine. Gross ignorance was often laced with thinly disguised homophobia or 'moral' judgment. For example, the then-Chief Constable of Greater Manchester Police, James Anderton, referred to people with AIDS 'swirling about in a human cesspit of their own making'.

In some parts of southern Africa, HIV myths took on a new, even more horrific dimension. First, it was rumored that sex with a virgin could cure AIDS, leading to increasing rape. Then another rumor began to spread that having intercourse with a baby would cure the disease. In 2001, 11 babies under one year old were raped in South Africa.

By the mid-1980s, Western governments and charities had moved to allay unfounded fears and increase understanding of the disease. Between 1985-86 and 1992-93 the British Government allocated more than £73 million to the development of the national AIDS public education campaign. It has never spent as much on domestic AIDS-awareness since.

The principal message of the HIV-prevention movement was 'safe sex'. Besides total abstinence, there was only one sure-fire way to prevent infection. Neither the pill nor modern antibiotics offered any defense. Condoms provided the only real barrier protection.

By this time, latex condoms were cheap and widely available. With global HIV campaigns promoting them as the most reliable and effective way to avoid infection, their popularity soared. In the UK, the increasing promotion of abstinence and condom use had a profound effect on the nation's sexual health. Although most campaigns were targeted specifically at stopping the spread of HIV, they actually helped to reduce incidence of all sexually transmitted infections.

Following major HIV and pro-condom campaigns, gonorrhea diagnoses in England and Wales plummeted from around 50,000 in 1985 to just 18,000 in 1988 – and had dropped to a 20th-century low by the mid-1990s. Syphilis fell from around 1,500 annual cases in the mid-1980s to around 150 in the mid-1990s. More recently, the numbers have been rising again. By 2005, incidence of syphilis had shot back up to 2,807 cases. Reasons for this rise include condom fatigue (see p 113) and growing complacency about HIV infection in those countries where advanced medication is available.

Globally, HIV/AIDS stands alongside malaria and tuberculosis as one of the most deadly infectious diseases facing humanity. Today, there are around 40 million people living with HIV worldwide. Some 14,000 people become infected every day, and the vast majority of these infections are from sexual contact. In 2006, 4.3 million people were newly infected with HIV and 2.9 million people died from AIDS. It remains the leading cause of

HIV AROUND THE WORLD
(2005 REGIONAL FIGURES)

	People with HIV	% of world's HIV cases	New cases	AIDS deaths
Sub-Saharan Africa	25.8 m	64%	3.2 m	2.4 m
Asia	8.3 m	20.6%	1.1 m	521,000
Western Europe & North America	1.9 m	4.7%	65,000	30,000
Latin America	1.8 m	4.5%	200,000	66,000
Eastern Europe & Central Asia	1.6 m	4%	270,000	62,000
Australia, New Zealand & Pacific Islands	74,000	0.18%	8,200	3,600
North Africa & Middle East	510,000	1.2%	67,000	58,000
Caribbean	300,000	0.7%	30,000	24,000

death in sub-Saharan Africa and the fourth leading killer worldwide. There is still no cure.

HIV and poverty

HIV is not spread equally around the world. An incredible 95 per cent of all people with HIV/AIDS live in the developing world, in exactly those countries which have the fewest facilities and least available treatments to ease people's suffering.

Although the precise origins of AIDS in Africa remain unknown, it is clear that HIV spread from West Africa across to the Indian Ocean in the 1970s and 1980s. The virus then moved to the southern African countries, where it now affects the most people.

Today, 32 per cent of all people with HIV live in southern Africa and 34 per cent of total AIDS deaths occur there. Swaziland currently has the highest adult HIV prevalence in the world, with 38 per cent HIV-positive – that is almost 4 in every 10 people aged 15 to 49. For many years, its neighbor South Africa and Botswana topped the table. In 2001, the peak rate of infection among 21-25 year old South Africans was 43.1 per cent. In 2005, there were 1,000 new infections and 800 deaths every day.

As well as the loss of life, this tragedy is crippling

African countries emotionally and socially. In Zambia, roughly half the teachers trained each year are dying from AIDS. The number of children orphaned by AIDS in sub-Saharan Africa (12 million) is almost the same as the entire child population of the UK. Christian Aid reports that by 2010, 43 million children will have been orphaned by AIDS worldwide.

One reason for the devastating spread of AIDS in Africa is a comparatively slow reaction by governments and health organizations to the outbreak. The reasons

ONE CONTINENT: HIV IN AFRICA

◆ Africans account for more than 60 per cent of global infections.

◆ Sub-Saharan Africa is more heavily affected by HIV and AIDS than any other region of the world.

◆ An estimated 25.8 million people were living with HIV in sub-Saharan Africa at the end of 2005.

◆ Approximately 3.2 million additional people were infected with HIV in 2005.

◆ In the past year, Africa's AIDS epidemic has claimed the lives of an estimated 2.4 million people.

◆ More than 12 million children have been orphaned by AIDS.

◆ Since the beginning of the epidemic more than 15 million Africans have died from AIDS.

for this lie in poverty, religious and moral attitudes, and lack of education – but also in denial, as in the case of South Africa.

Stephen Lewis, UN Special Envoy for HIV/AIDS in Africa, stated in 2006 that: 'South Africa is the unkindest

---

GARLIC AND BEETROOT

The AIDS epidemic claims nearly 1,000 lives a day in South Africa. UNAIDS, the UN's program on combating HIV/AIDS, states that almost 11 per cent of the population are HIV-positive. Yet at the 2006 International AIDS Conference in Canada, the South African stall caused many AIDS experts to shake their heads in disbelief. Alongside a display of anti-retroviral drugs (ARVs) stood a heap of lemons, garlic and beetroots. South Africa's health minister, Manto Tshabalala-Msimang provoked international outrage when she claimed that these vegetables were a serious alternative to drug treatments in combating AIDS.

Deputy-President Phumzile Mlambo-Ngcuka took control of national AIDS policy in September and recently Tshabalala-Msimang has been hospitalized. The Government has finally responded to pressure from groups such as the Treatment Action Campaign and announced a change in direction, promising for the first time to set targets for cutting rates of infection and getting anti-AIDS drugs to all who need them by 2010. ◆

---

cut of all. It is the only country in Africa... whose government is still obtuse, dilatory and negligent about rolling out treatment. It is the only country in Africa whose government continues to propound theories more worthy of a lunatic fringe than of a concerned and compassionate state.'

South African President Mbeki has consistently refused to acknowledge that HIV is the cause of AIDS; he argues that HIV is just one factor amongst many that might contribute to deaths resulting from immunodeficiency, alongside others such as poverty and poor nutrition.

Medical anthropologist Dr Suzanne Leclerc-Madlala says that more than anywhere else in the world, the advent of AIDS in Africa was met with apathy, or what some researchers have called 'an under-reaction'. This came in direct contrast to responses in Europe, the US, parts of Asia and Australia, for example, where serious discussion of HIV/AIDS produced marked sexual behavioral change.

In Thailand, for example, the first evidence of the arrival of AIDS saw a rapid dwindling of clients at brothels, and many were forced to close due to lack of business. The scenario was similar for both North America and parts of South America, where education campaigns were given priority. 'These reactions occurred as a response to HIV levels that were a fraction of those found in Africa,' says Dr Leclerc-Madlala, 'Yet no such reaction was recorded for Africa.'

Lack of education can have a dramatic effect on HIV incidence. Research by the Nelson Mandela Foundation found that 35 per cent of 12-14 year olds in South Africa thought that sex with a virgin could cure AIDS. There are many other persistent myths held throughout the countries with the highest prevalence of HIV cases. This ignorance is frequently exacerbated due to poor schooling provision and a family's need for children to start work at a young age. It can have potentially deadly consequences.

Before the outbreak of HIV, condom use was rare in many parts of Africa. Since the 1980s, there have been efforts to change behavior and increase supply to the areas most affected by the virus.

The business of condoms

The question of whether condoms are ordinary retail commodities or essential medical supplies has affected the nature and scope of condom distribution worldwide. For many people, the outbreak of HIV/AIDS, and its prevalence in poor, developing nations, has blurred the boundaries. Globally, the condom industry is a multi-billion dollar market. In 2005, the US market stood at $398 million, up 2.8 per cent from 2004. Of the global condom export market the EU currently commands a 40-per-cent market share, while Thailand has 15 per cent. Other major condom exporters include the US, India and Malaysia.

Given that Thailand is the world's top rubber producer, it should perhaps come as no surprise that it is also the number one exporter of condoms. Every year, about three billion condoms are produced in Thailand, more than 75 per cent destined for export. In 2007, its exports are predicted to be worth more than $55 million. Nevertheless, Thailand still imports about $1 million of condoms a year, mainly the top-end ultra-thin or exotically flavored varieties.

In those developing countries where governments have both the resources and political will to promote condom use, millions are routinely given out free as 'social marketing' exercises. Population Action International reports that the governments of South Africa and Botswana, two of the wealthiest and hardest-hit countries in sub-Saharan Africa, provide 'the vast majority of condoms for distribution in their countries

EASY AS ABC

In January 2003, President George W Bush initiated the Presidential Emergency Plan for AIDS Relief (PEPFAR) with an HIV-prevention program built around the motto, 'ABC'. This was likely based on a safe sex message reportedly first adopted by the Botswana Government in the late 1990s. Promoted on billboards around the country were the words:

A – Abstain from sex

B – Be faithful to one monogamous partner

C – use Condoms

This 'ABC' message has enjoyed much success, most notably in Uganda. Critics of US international development policy, however, note that too much emphasis is placed on A and B over C (see page 71). Some AIDS campaigners have even criticized the entire ABC model as ill-conceived and counterproductive. They argue that a much larger alphabet is required, such as another C for male circumcision, D for diaphragm, all the way through to I for immunity by vaccines. ◆

through the public sector and social marketing'. In 2000, they purchased 290 million and 12 million condoms, respectively. In comparison, all donors combined provided 400 million condoms to the whole of sub-Saharan Africa in that year.

Like several other Asian nations, the Indian Government has also long promoted condom use for family planning. In 2000, government social marketing programs were responsible for distributing 450 million condoms nationwide. This level of public sector support varies enormously from one country to another. While Brazil, China and India are self-sufficient in condoms, many other Asian and African countries are hugely reliant on outside donations. Where donor support does not meet condom requirements, poor countries often have to pay for imported condoms with funds needed for food, medicine and other necessities.

UNAIDS, the joint UN Program on combating HIV/AIDS, has estimated that 13 billion condoms are needed every year to help halt the spread of HIV and other sexually transmitted infections. The reality falls short. In 2004, the UN Population Fund (UNFPA) and social marketing organizations together provided 2.1 billion condoms. UNFPA reports that in that same year, sub-Saharan Africa – the region with greatest HIV prevalence and the largest share of donor support – received only 10 condoms per man of reproductive age. Although this is double the amount provided in 2001, it still falls well below what is actually required.

The need for promotion and distribution of condoms still far outstrips the resources committed. An estimated

9.9 billion condoms were needed in 2002 to significantly reduce the rate of HIV infection and prevalence in the developing world and eastern Europe. Donors provided 2.5 billion condoms that year, up from 950 million in 2000. UNFPA predicts that at least 18.6 billion condoms will be needed by 2015. In one country, Uganda, 120-150 million condoms were needed in 2005, but less than 40 million were provided.

While condom use and distribution has increased in many African countries south of the Sahara in the last decade, donor provision has not met the demand required to meaningfully combat the HIV/AIDS epidemic. This is even more disappointing given the very low price of condoms on the global market. Today, the average international price is just three cents per male condom, which includes the costs of sampling, testing and shipping.

Private companies generally have only a small presence where HIV is most prevalent. In sub-Saharan Africa, there are few commercial opportunities, and therefore little interest. This contrasts with other Majority World countries in Asia and Latin America, notably Brazil, the Philippines and Indonesia, where there is money to be made. Population Action International reports that in Brazil, 350 million male condoms were sold through the commercial sector in 2000, three times the number distributed by the Government.

ESTIMATED CONDOM REQUIREMENTS COMPARED WITH ACTUAL DONOR SUPPORT IN 2000 ($ MILLIONS)

Region	Estimated family planning condom needs	Estimated STI*/HIV prevention condom needs	Total condom needs	Actual donor supply (2000)	Gap between need and supply
Africa	5.0	33.0	38.0	22.3	15.7
Asia	42.7	135.0	177.7	17.5	160.2
Arab States & Europe	12.6	34.0	47.6	1.1	46.5
Latin America & Caribbean	14.5	37.0	51.5	5.0	46.5
Totals	74.8	239.0	314.8	45.9	268.9**

*Sexually transmitted infection
** Some of the $268.9 million gap may in fact be covered by various other means including: more people buying condoms in the private sector, and/or increased spending by governments.

Global Estimates of Contraceptive Commodities and Condoms for STI/HIV Prevention 2000-2015, UNFPA, 2002.

A global legacy

Death tolls are only one measure of the tragic impact of HIV. There are also highly distressing implications for the future economic survival and social cohesion of many poor countries. Currently almost half of all new HIV infections occur among people under 25. The majority of these infected people living in the Majority World, who are largely unable to access expensive, life-prolonging treatment and care, will die by the age of 35.

Beyond this direct human tragedy lies a further catastrophe in the making. The potential loss of generations of people in their most productive years will have a devastating effect on developing countries. By 2020, Botswana, for example, is projected to have fewer people aged 40-50 than aged 60-80. In other words, a smaller number of adults of productive working age will be supporting greater numbers of children and older people. This will have a crippling effect on the country's economic and social fabric. In addition, where both HIV-infected parents die from AIDS, the very young and the very old increasingly have to take care of each other.

In South Africa alone, it has been estimated that $22 billion will have been wiped off the economy by 2010 because of AIDS. In Zambia, experts predict that companies will be spending the equivalent of a fifth of their salary bills on AIDS-related benefits. Beside issues of cost, availability and the consequences of not using condoms, however, is the backdrop of religion and moral views about contraception.

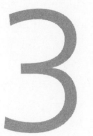# 3

Guilty pleasures

Ever since Fallopio's first devices to ward off syphilis, the humble sheath has suffered many negative social and cultural connotations. Initially, only wealthy philanderers would have required or afforded condoms – and it has taken a long time to change the perception that they are not for regular, decent people. Condoms may have become cheaper, more available and gradually less stigmatized over the centuries, but their popularity still remains tightly linked to prevailing attitudes towards sex, religion and other cultural beliefs.

Historically, they have faced a series of cultural challenges. In Victorian England for example sex was supposedly taboo. At a time when curvaceous table legs were being covered up lest they arouse unwanted sexual desires, condoms were hardly acceptable in polite conversation – and not between the bed-sheets either.

One of the most frequent early arguments *against*

SANGER'S PLIGHT

A contemporary of British birth-control pioneer Marie Stopes, the American socialist Margaret Sanger opened the first sexual clinic and advice center in the US in 1916. In outright defiance of the Comstock Law (see p 55), she promoted contraception as a means of female liberation. Her forthright opinions on marriage ('the most degenerate influence on the social order') and women's rights won her many enemies. But she remained a powerful voice in the birth-control movement – especially among poor women, who had been kept largely ignorant of contraceptive methods. The founder of advice organization Planned Parenthood (which still lives on as offshoots of the US Family Planning Associations), she was responsible for offering women information and advice on contraceptives. Sanger was adamant that women should not need permission from their doctor, partner or parents.

In early 1914, she published her first issue of *The Woman Rebel*, a magazine for radical feminists. Three issues were banned for promoting the use of contraception, and in August of that year Sanger was indicted on nine charges of violating the Comstock Law.

---

condoms was that within wholesome, monogamous relationships, they were simply unnecessary. The logic went that since only sexual scoundrels would require them, their use was hardly to be condoned. At first,

To avoid prosecution, she fled the country to England under the assumed name, Bertha Watson. From abroad, she ordered 100,000 copies of a new pamphlet promoting contraception, entitled *Family Limitation*, to be distributed in the US.

While in England, she met Marie Stopes. They shared very similar opinions on both birth control and eugenics, and began working together. But their relationship would cool over differences in directions: Sanger was interested in advocating sexual rights for all women, while Stopes concentrated mainly on married couples.

When Sanger returned to the US, she was arrested, fined

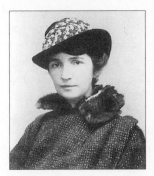

and imprisoned for distributing information on birth control. While this ruling was overturned on appeal, the prohibition of mailing anything to do with birth control was not repealed for another 18 years. Indeed, one of the last of the Comstock Laws was not overturned in the US until 1966, the year of Sanger's death. ◆

the backlash was not especially organized. But as the condom industry began to flourish, so too an increasingly united self-appointed band of 'moral guardians' began to emerge.

Moral minority

In the US, one of the first voices of resistance belonged to book-burning prude Anthony Comstock, head of the

POPULATION DECLINE

Falling birth rates frequently explain one-off reactions against condoms over the centuries. As birth-control centers were opening in Britain in the early 20th century, other countries were far less keen to promote contraception. As a result of World War One France faced a severe fall in population, and in particular a shortage of young men. As a result, contraception was banned in 1920. Curiously, this policy was also extended to its colonies and mandates, such as Syria, whose government had no desire to restrict birth control. In France, many young women faced the unpleasant prospect of having to reproduce with the older men who had been left behind when the younger men went off to fight.

Hitler's plans for national expansion also required a burgeoning German population. In 1933, the Nazis prohibited all contraception. But population decline in Germany had already

New York Society for the Prevention of Vice. In 1873, Comstock successfully persuaded the US Congress to pass the Comstock Law, which made it illegal to send any 'obscene, lewd, and/or lascivious' materials through the post. This included all contraceptive devices or information about contraception. Comstock believed all forms of birth control to be immoral and was bullish in his determination to stamp down on those 'depraved'

been a concern in the 1920s when contraceptive advertising had been banned, albeit without much success.

In Italy, another country to suffer a fall in population numbers in the 20th century, the advertising ban on contraception was only lifted in 1971. Many countries have discouraged contraception when they needed more people, especially troops.

Japan has also clamped down on the condom. The Japanese Government had first banned condoms and abortion (except in women with life-threatening medical complications) in the 1870s. Even well into the 20th century, the Government was cool on the idea of condom promotion. In 1922, US birth-control pioneer Margaret Sanger was invited by friends to stay with them in Japan. When she arrived at Yokohama, however, the Japanese Government refused to allow her to enter the country. Only after promising not to give any lectures on birth control during her visit was she finally given permission to land. ◆

souls who continued to promote them.

The American Social Hygiene Association was also active in the early 20th century, campaigning to prohibit condoms. Its members argued that anyone who contracted a venereal disease deserved to suffer the consequences. Organizations such as this were responsible for the fact that US soldiers (unlike their European allies) went without condoms in World War One – and often returned home riddled with STDs. Nevertheless, the anti-birth-control lobby went from strength to strength. For almost 100 years, condoms could only be sold in the US with the warning 'For disease prevention only'.

By World War Two, US thinking on condoms had changed. In an attempt to avert the same sexual health problems experienced by the military in World War One, condoms were promoted heavily. For the 'morally upstanding' followers of Comstock, it was a global disgrace. And as the condom's popularity and acceptance continued to boom after the War, the prophylactics presented an even bigger threat, especially to those fundamentally opposed to birth control on religious grounds. Across the world, men of the cloth were beginning to sharpen their knives against the sheath.

Catholics and condoms

It is perhaps astonishing that a pocket-sized piece of rubber could provoke such a ferocious reaction from the Catholic Church. For many centuries, condoms were simply not sufficiently popular to be considered much of a challenge to official church dogma. But as they became more widely available and publicly accepted, so Catholic leaders began to tackle the issue head-on.

According to official doctrine, there can be no barrier between sex and procreation. This argument has its roots in the Old Testament. In Genesis, Onan incurred God's wrath by using *coitus interruptus* ('spilling his seed on the ground') rather than impregnating his sister-in-law after the death of his brother. Since then, many Christians (and Jews) have considered it a sin to ejaculate if the sperm will die. This rules out withdrawal, masturbation, intra-vaginal contraceptives... and condoms.

While possibly incompatible with a man's basic sexual urges, this doctrine appeared to pose only the most modest *physical* harm when it was enshrined by Pope Pius XI in 1930. In *Casti Connubii*, which set out the duties of Christian marriage, the Vatican declared that artificial contraception was shameful and immoral. Devout Catholics were therefore banned from all methods of contraception except for sexual intercourse during the so-called 'safe' period of a woman's menstrual cycle, a practice often dubbed 'Vatican Roulette'.

Thanks to the arrival of effective antibiotics to deal with STIs, the 'only' unwelcome outcome of unprotected sex was an 'unwanted' pregnancy – and to deem any baby as unwanted is hard for most women. In this way, with the Church's doctrine of no sex before marriage and lifelong fidelity, condoms were essentially seen as an irrelevance.

By the mid-1960s, sexual attitudes in the West were changing. For the 'summer of love' generation, sex was no longer taboo. Thanks to the pill, women were taking greater control over their sex lives and procreation. For many, this era presented a golden opportunity for the Vatican to reflect modern thinking and formally accept contraception. Instead, it published the *Humanae Vitai*, a landmark document for the Catholic Church, which reaffirmed the Church's prohibition of contraception.

In the 1980s, the Church had another chance to soften its line. By this time, the devastating effects of HIV/AIDS had persuaded even many previously conservative religious thinkers that the church must relax its stance on condoms. Without a change in the official Catholic position, millions of people would be risking a very different and deadlier game of Vatican Roulette. But again there was to be no compromise.

In 1987, Pope John Paul II and Cardinal Joseph Ratzinger, now the incumbent Pope Benedict XVI, together published the *Donum Vitae*, which declared that the Church could *never* agree to the use of contraceptives by men and women who were not married or who were in homosexual relationships. No mention was made of married couples.

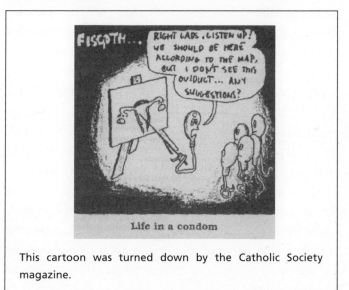

Life in a condom

This cartoon was turned down by the Catholic Society magazine.

This series of hard-line Vatican publications has condemned millions of god-fearing people to a perilous life without condoms. In the fight against HIV/AIDS, and in Catholic parts of Africa and Latin America especially, where HIV/AIDS education and treatments have been directly affected as a result, it has had horrific consequences.

Today, there are approximately 150 million Catholics in Africa. Between 1900 and 2000, their numbers rose from 1.9 million to 130 million. As seen, the continent also accounts for more than 60 per cent of all global HIV infections. More than 15 million Africans have died from AIDS since the start of the epidemic. It is impossible to know how many of these lives would have been spared if their faith had allowed them to use condoms.

UNAIDS estimates that there are 1.6 million people living with HIV/AIDS in Latin America. It is estimated that 600 to 700 people in Latin America and the Caribbean are infected with the virus every day – about one person every two minutes. It is no coincidence that the population of Latin America is predominantly Catholic. Due to the Vatican's refusal to acknowledge any safe sex practices besides abstinence, education about contraceptives and condom use has remained very low.

Not only has the Vatican instructed Catholics not to use condoms, it has also spread untruths about their effectiveness. In 2003, the BBC reported that the Catholic Church had been telling people in countries stricken by AIDS to shun condoms because they have tiny holes in them through which HIV can pass. In the BBC *Panorama* program 'Sex and the Holy City', the president of the Vatican's Pontifical Council for the Family, Cardinal Alfonso Lopez Trujillo, said: 'The AIDS virus is roughly 450 times smaller than the spermatozoon. The spermatozoon can easily pass through the "net" that is formed by the condom.'

Catholic leaders have repeated these erroneous claims throughout the world. And while the UN immediately rejected Trujillo's outburst as scientifically incorrect, much damage had already been done. Given the influence of the Catholic Church in many developing countries, where HIV is most prevalent, it has been the equivalent of a death sentence. In the Philippines, for example, the Church is a very powerful force in politics. Since 2004, the Government has prevented promotion and distribution of condoms, and many local authorities have banned health workers from even discussing them. The Philippine National AIDS Council now describes the HIV epidemic as 'hidden and growing', while Human Rights Watch has described the situation as a 'a social time bomb'.

The responsibility for these policies goes all the way to the top. Speaking to an audience of bishops from South Africa, Swaziland, Botswana, Namibia and Lesotho in 2005, Pope Benedict said of AIDS: 'It's a great concern that the fabric of African life, its very source of hope and stability, is threatened by divorce, abortion, prostitution, human trafficking and a contraception mentality.' In another speech later that same year, he listed several ways to combat the spread of HIV, including chastity, fidelity in marriage and antipoverty efforts. He did not mention condoms once.

Nevertheless, there are signs that the official Catholic stance on condoms might one day be relaxed. In recent years, there have been a growing number of dissenting voices from within the Church. Religious organizations, such as Catholics for a Free Choice, believe that condoms should be accepted as a way to fight AIDS. Cardinal Carlo Maria Martini, the retired Archbishop of Milan, has said that condoms could be a 'lesser evil' when used in the context of marriage to prevent the spread of HIV. Other senior clergy have argued that not promoting condoms is tantamount to breaking one of the Ten Commandments:

'Thou shalt not kill'.

There are also reports of believers simply ignoring official doctrine. In El Salvador, for example, where only four per cent of women use contraceptives the first time they have sex, *New York Times* writer Nicholas Kristof reported that the grassroots Church is defying the Vatican and teaching people about condoms and AIDS. 'Certainly, God does not want us to kill each other,' said one Sister, who works with AIDS patients. 'You've got to do something.'

It has even been rumored that Pope Benedict has requested a report on whether it might be acceptable for Catholics to use condoms in one circumstance: to protect life inside a marriage when one partner is infected with HIV or sick with AIDS. After all, the original *Donum Vitae* said nothing about condom use between married couples. While this would be a genuinely meaningful commitment (married couples actually top infection rates in many developing countries), it would still place millions of unmarried people's lives at unnecessary risk.

Ironically, the Catholic Church plays a huge role in caring for those people affected by HIV and AIDS in many parts of the world. Indeed, it is estimated that some 25 per cent of all AIDS care worldwide is provided by Catholic-related groups. How tragic that the Vatican's anti-condom propaganda is only exacerbating the AIDS crisis, and increasing the unnecessary suffering of millions worldwide.

God's wrath

While the Catholic Church is well known for its rejection of all artificial contraception, many of the world's other major religions also have an uneasy relationship with condoms. Most faiths embrace both orthodox believers and more liberal adherents. Orthodox Jews, for example, also refer back to Genesis for their position on contraception. In other words, condoms are unallowable because they contradict the commandment against 'killing the seed'. Reform Jews, however, are less strict on this point, while liberal Jews fully accept condom use.

In Islam, condom use is permitted so long as it is between a married heterosexual couple and there is a valid reason for birth control, such as the wife's poor health to avoid pregnancy, or 'personal reasons dictated by conscience'.

In the booklet 'Islam's Attitude Towards Family Planning', for instance, the Arab Republic of Egypt concluded any method that has the same purpose as *azl* (*coitus interruptus*) and does not induce permanent sterility is acceptable for Muslims.

But it is important to remember that a key precept here is no sex before marriage. In other words, condoms are only acceptable within monogamous married relationships in order to space out children.

One of the most common (and misguided) arguments against condom promotion is that it encourages promiscuity. For many 'moral guardians' in society, this equation (more education = more intercourse) is reason enough to oppose any push on contraception. While factually incorrect, this has not stopped many hard-line religious thinkers and politicians from decrying or willfully ignoring the importance of the condom. Al-Qaeda leader Osama Bin Laden, President George W Bush and Pope Benedict make unlikely bedfellows in this fight against condoms.

Certainly, this equation also explains why Muslim clerics from 25 African countries failed to reach an agreement on the use of condoms for preventing HIV/AIDS at a meeting in Zanzibar in December 2006. In certain fundamentalist Islamic states, Sharia law has been cited as grounds to invoke a total ban on condoms. Indeed, in 2003, a powerful Somali Muslim group banned selling or using condoms in Somalia. The punishments for violation include flogging.

There has been no such crackdown in Buddhist countries, but followers are reluctant to tamper with the natural development of life. This means no interference is allowed once the sperm and egg fuse. Buddhists are therefore strongly opposed to abortion, but generally accept condoms and the pill.

Sikhs believe in monogamy and great importance is attached to sexual morality. However, condoms have never been banned and attitudes to birth control have moved with the times. Today, contraception is an acceptable practice within Sikhism.

Hinduism has evolved over thousands of years, and has a huge variety of wide-ranging and complex teachings about all aspects of human life. When it comes to contraception, all methods are allowed.

The politics of condoms

The impact of religious doctrine on condom promotion, distribution and use often depends on the influence of a particular religion on the prevailing political landscape. In the US, for example, the Christian-Right Republican government under George W Bush has had an influence

> 'It seems to me the contraceptive message sends a
> contradictory message. It tends to undermine the message
> of abstinence.'
>
> US presidential candidate George W Bush in 1999.

on everything from how sex and contraception are taught
in schools at home to how HIV-prevention programs are
carried out abroad.

In 2002, US writer Doug Ireland referred to Bush's 'war
on the condom'. He noted that at the UN Special Session
on Children in New York that year, the US delegation
joined with Iran and Saddam Hussein's Iraq to demand
the removal of all references to 'reproductive health
services and education'. This attitude also explained why
between 1993 and 2003, the number of condoms the
US contributed worldwide fell from 800 million to 300
million.

The US delegation at the 2002 UN-sponsored Asian
and Pacific Population Conference again attempted (and
failed) to delete endorsement of 'consistent condom use'
as a means of preventing HIV infection. Once again,
they equated condom promotion with promiscuity. In
fact, numerous scientific studies prove that proper sex
education actually delays the onset of sexual activity.

That year, the US spent $500 million on abstinence-only programs – more than twice as much as it donated to the UN-backed Global Fund to fight AIDS, TB and Malaria, which supports condom promotion.

Ireland reports that since taking office, Bush has 'stacked the President's Advisory Council on HIV & AIDS with abstinence-only advocates and condom opponents', and increased the amount the US spends on abstinence-only domestic sex education by 33 per cent. Indeed in 2004, one third of all US federal HIV-education money was allocated to abstinence-only programs, almost universally to

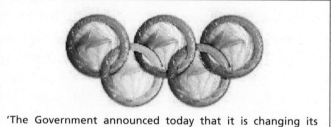

'The Government announced today that it is changing its emblem to a condom because it more clearly reflects the government's political stance. A condom stands up to inflation, halts production, destroys the next generation, protects a bunch of pricks, and gives you a sense of security while you're actually being screwed.'

DAMN, it just doesn't get more accurate than that!!!

Christian groups as part of Bush's 'faith-based initiatives' (no Jewish or Muslim groups receive any funds).

Because of the Bush Administration's attitude, US citizens today are finding it increasingly difficult to find information about responsible sexual practice. Meanwhile, more and more children are not being told about the single most effective method of preventing HIV. Global watchdog organization Human Rights Watch quotes a Texas school official as saying, 'We don't discuss condom use, except to say that condoms don't work'.

Further afield, US policy is directly undermining the global fight against HIV/AIDS. In an attempt to secure more US funding, many Majority World governments have begun to publicly endorse abstinence and condemn contraception. In May 2004, President Yoweri Museveni of Uganda, who had long supported condoms as part of a successful prevention strategy, caused outrage by declaring that they should only be provided to sex-workers. Earlier that same year, the Government in Zambia, a country with one of the highest incidences of HIV in the world, reportedly banned distributing condoms in schools, claiming they spread promiscuity among youth.

Writing in British newspaper *The Guardian*, Stephen

Lewis, the UN special envoy for HIV/AIDS in Africa, reiterated that US cuts in funding for condoms and an emphasis on promoting abstinence had contributed to a shortage of condoms in Uganda, one of the few African countries which had succeeded in reducing its infection rate. 'There is no doubt in my mind that the condom crisis in Uganda is being driven by [US policies],' he said. 'To impose a dogma-driven policy that is fundamentally flawed is doing damage to Africa.'

In 2006, Reuters reported that USAID, the largest provider of contraceptives for the past 30 years to the Philippines, has stopped supplying condoms and plans to end the rest of its contraceptive donation program by 2008. Dr Zahidul Huque of the UN's Population Fund (UNFPA) said private businesses in the Philippines were not ready to take up where USAID was leaving off for fear of a negative reaction from the Church. 'USAID is pulling out without preparing the country,' Huque said. In the absence of a government push to tackle population growth, charities and local medical professionals are now trying to fill the gap.

Another damaging effect of the US 'pro-abstinence only' policy is to isolate and weaken those family planning organizations that support a woman's right to abortion or contraception, or that simply dare to mention them in counseling sessions. Indeed, abortion centers have long been a target of US economic sanctions. The Mexico City Policy, often called the 'Global Gag Rule', was introduced by President Reagan as far back as 1984. This states that no US family planning assistance can be provided to foreign NGOs which use funding from any other source to perform abortions, with very few exceptions. Abolished by President Clinton, it was immediately reintroduced by George W Bush when he took office in January 2001.

Given that the US is the largest donor of reproductive

HARD CASH

What one million dollars in commodity support* for contraceptives can do:

◆ Save the lives of 800 women and 11,000 infants

◆ Prevent some 14,000 additional deaths of children under 5

◆ Avert 360,000 unwanted pregnancies

◆ Prevent 150,000 additional induced abortions

*Commodity support covers not only the supply of commodities but also resources for their purchase, technical assistance and provider support necessary to ensure that the commodities are well used, and provide support to developing countries to enhance their own commodity supply systems.

UNFPA

health funds globally, this rule has had significant effects throughout the world. Many abortion clinics doubling as contraceptive advice centers are increasingly forced to shut, and so too the condom message is being silenced.

Pleasure principle

While religious leaders and conservative politicians publicly condemn the condom, arguably its biggest critics come from within the bedroom. Birth control and disease prevention issues aside, studies show that men and women resoundingly prefer sex without condoms. The most common explanation is that they reduce the pleasure of sexual intercourse.

Despite the modern advances in ultra-thin latex, a condom is still an artificial barrier between two lovers' bodies. For many people, this results in reduced sensation, less intimacy and a weaker orgasm. In many parts of Africa, the practice of condom-free intercourse is nicknamed 'eating the sweetie without the wrapper'.

The reduced sensitivity is largely due to the transfer

'Using condoms is like listening to a symphony with cotton wool in your ears.'

Anon.

HOW SAFE IS SAFE?

Modern latex condoms undergo numerous stringent safety checks. First, each one is tested for pinholes using an electronic test. Here, the condom is pulled over a metal form called a mandrel and placed within an intense electrical field. Because rubber does not conduct electricity, no electricity should reach the metal mandrel under the condom. If it does, this indicates the presence of a pinhole. Any condom failing this test is discarded (machines discard the failures automatically). Additional checks include an air burst test. Here, the condom is filled with air until it pops. The air pressure and amount of air inside the condom are measured at the time the condom breaks. If these numbers are too low in more than 1.5 out of 100 condoms, the entire lot is discarded.

Thanks to these safety measures, and with consistent and correct use, the World Health Organization reports that condoms ensure a 'near-zero risk' of HIV. Studies on couples where one partner is infected show that 'with consistent condom use, HIV infection rates for the uninfected partner are below one per cent a year'. ◆

of heat. In unprotected sex, there is a direct transfer of heat from the penis to the vagina, which can create more intimacy and arousal. Latex slows this heat transfer, creating a cooler, less natural feel. For many people, the smell of the material is also a major turn-off.

Putting on a condom can often be an inconvenience too. While this can be introduced into foreplay, stopping to find and then put on a condom is often an unwanted or even embarrassing interruption of an otherwise very natural act. Many couples talk of condoms 'killing the moment'.

It is impossible to know how many people refuse to use condoms because of purely aesthetic reasons, but it is likely to have a huge effect on the number of people practicing safe sex at any one time.

Culture clash

Aesthetic considerations often feed into wider societal and cultural bias against the condom. In 2006, Reuters reported that in the Philippines, macho culture and myths about side-effects from condoms (used by only an estimated 1.9 per cent of married couples), and also about vasectomies mean that contraception in the country is seen as the woman's problem.

Indeed, arguably the most fundamental social factor working against condom use is gender inequality. Despite men's culpability in not providing better protection for themselves and their partners, they too can be under pressure to ignore contraception. Some women also may regard condom-free sex as a sign of intimacy and trust. If their man insists on using protection, it can be seen as a slight – suggesting she is unclean or simply a casual sex partner.

There are other factors, however, which affect contraceptive use. In their 2001 research paper on condom use among sex-workers in Nigeria, Muyiwa Oladosu and Olaronke Lapido conclude that 'the social context of gender relations, poverty, poor administration of brothels and government laws and regulations (all) discourage condom use'.

They argue that sex-workers' ability to ask their clients

to use condoms is 'negatively affected by the male-dominant Nigerian society that gives men undue influence over decision-making on important issues'. These gender dynamics make it possible for clients who do not want to use condoms to more easily convince sex-workers to have unsafe sex. The men in question are likely to behave the same way with any partners or wives – and may beat women who do not acquiesce.

As a result, statistics on condom use can often appear shockingly low. In his socio-cultural study of condom use within marriage in rural Lebanon, Professor Andrzej Kulczycki concluded that only seven per cent of married couples used condoms, despite growing awareness of STDs and HIV. Explanations for this behavior included 'various encumbering beliefs, reduced sexual pleasure, adverse experiences, gender-related fears and tensions, and a residual social stigma attached to condoms'. Many women simply have no choice in the matter. Where this is the case, they may inadvertently internalize presiding male views about condoms.

The mere act of covering their manhood is another turn-off for many men. This can be reflected in the ultra-macho names adopted by many of the world's leading condom brands, such as Trojan in the US, and Sheba and

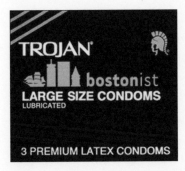

Simba in Africa. Another social stigma harks back to the condom's earliest incarnation. In many parts of the world, it is still considered suitable only for sexually promiscuous men. And whatever the reality, many men like to think that they personally are not promiscuous.

Size matters

Condom size is also a delicate issue. Some African communities, for example, have criticized Japanese condoms for being too small. In India, many men have reportedly had the opposite problem. In 2006, a survey showed that condoms made according to international sizes are too large for some Indian men. This is a serious issue because about one in every five times a condom is used in India it either falls off or tears, an extremely high failure rate. The poor fit may also put Indian men off using condoms at all. And even a hint of just such a possibility can be used to justify not wearing them.

Underlying many of these cultural problems is the

lack of mature discussion about sex and contraception. Where talking about sex remains largely taboo, especially because of prevailing social or religious beliefs, education about contraception is likely to be very poor.

This attitude affects many Western countries, too. In the UK, the most complained-about advertisement ever remains the 1995 poster for the British Safety Council. It featured a picture of the Pope with the legend: 'Thou shalt always wear a condom.'

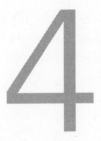

Sex change

'You have to say, I am going to take care of myself. If this guy is not going to use a condom, I'm not going to get into that situation.'

KIM CATTRALL, *SEX IN THE CITY*.

Ever since the condom's first incarnation, the decision to use or not use one has typically rested with the wearer. Only in the last few decades, and in a relatively small number of cultures, have women had much say about condoms – and had other recourses if their wishes are refused.

Why? The major reason for women's historically distanced relationship from the condom is their second-class status in many global cultures. If they are excluded from *all* important decisions in society, it is no surprise if they also have little say about what goes on in the bedroom. Indeed, where this reality is deeply internalized it may not occur to a woman that she is even entitled to ask her partner to use a condom. And if she does, there may be unpleasant consequences such as anger and violence.

Women and the condom

In a marriage, a woman can risk accusations of infidelity or even violence if she insists on condoms. As a result, she may deliberately remain apparently ignorant of the facts of sexuality and HIV/AIDS because she is not 'supposed' to be sexually knowledgeable. In Kenya, wives have cited the inability to talk to their husbands about condoms lest they be accused of learning about sex in extramarital affairs. Ironically, many men may also remain ignorant about HIV/AIDS because they *are* 'supposed' to be sexually all-knowing.

The very concept of monogamous life-partnerships or marriages presents another problem for many women. Where local culture dictates that a man's sexual appetites are fulfilled whenever and wherever he so wishes, his wife at home runs a much greater risk of contracting STDs or HIV – especially if she is also in no position to insist on using contraception.

Culture clash

In 2004, UNICEF encountered deepening flaws in Uganda's once successful ABC (Abstinence, Being faithful and Condoms) message. The agency reported that women were increasingly being 'coerced into unprotected sex by partners [whose] desire to "eat the sweet without the wrapper" [made] a mockery out of the idea of condom use'.

Some women, however, are equally uncomfortable with condoms – regardless of the consequences. According to US-based Johns Hopkins Bloomberg School of Public Health, in many African and Asian communities, women who believe that their husbands are infected with HIV still agree to have unprotected sex with them because having children is important to their status in the family and community. It is however questionable whether they would have the choice to refuse anyway. The report added that in Nepal, concerns about having 'good character' also prevented many women from asking the man to use condoms.

Ironically, marriage and fidelity often provide little protection to women anyway. Numerous studies have shown that many infected women are faithful to their husbands. In Cambodia and Thailand, which have the highest HIV prevalence in Asia and the Pacific, the bulk of new infections occur through marital sex, invariably from husband to wife. Male infidelity with sex-workers is predominantly to blame.

Condom use depends on a variety of other cultural factors too. In 1999, the US weekly *Village Voice* reported that dry, abrasive vaginas are seen as desirable in sexual intercourse in many southern African cultures. A common perception is that loose, slippery vaginas are evidence of infidelity, while dry vaginas are tighter and make the man feel bigger. Dryness, however, not only causes great pain for the woman, it also drastically increases the risk of contracting HIV through the lacerations that are caused in the vaginal tissue. It also means a lack of natural antiseptic present in vaginal juices and higher incidence of condom breakage. Because of this cultural attitude, it is even harder for a woman to use an effective spermicide as this would also act as a lubricant.

Within all these cultural contexts, the common thread is the lack of male responsibility. Given that safe sex needs a man not only to agree in principle to condoms, but also to actually put one on, a woman is at an immediate disadvantage. This explains why only an average of 4.9 per cent of married women of reproductive age worldwide use condoms. In developing countries, the figure is even lower.

Contraceptive choice

As discussed earlier, the idea of blocking the cervix to prevent pregnancy is thousands of years old. Crude pessaries, such as honey, crocodile-dung and lemon halves, have been used as methods of birth control since time immemorial. Only at the beginning of the 20th century, however, did scientists begin to develop pessaries that actually extended into the uterus. While early incarnations, which used catgut as a thread, led to high infection rates, this primitive device was nonetheless very popular during the First World War.

Since then, there have been many technological advancements in female contraception and a much greater choice. Before the 1960s, the cervical cap, a thimble-shaped device, was the most widely used contraceptive method in western Europe. In the US, women preferred the diaphragm, which has a flexible rim and sits less tightly over the cervix; by 1940, one third of all US married couples were using this contraceptive device. But thanks to new and more convenient birth-control methods, by 1965 only 10 per cent of US married

CONDOM • TRIGGER ISSUES

couples were using a diaphragm for contraception. That number has continued to fall, and in 2002 only 0.2 per cent of American women were using a diaphragm as their primary method of contraception.

The mid-20th century also saw the invention of the intra-uterine device (IUD). A piece of metal or plastic inserted into the woman's uterus from the vagina by a physician, this stops pregnancy by preventing the egg

TAKING CONTROL

Arguably the most important pill to be popped during the 1960s was the contraceptive variety. Invented by American biologist Dr Gregory Pincus, the new oral birth-control tablet had been first tested in Puerto Rico in 1956 and found to successfully suppress ovulation. Hailed as one of the most significant medical advances of the 20th century, take-up was rapid. By 1967, the number of users was in excess of 12.5 million worldwide. By 1984, this figure had risen to between 50 and 80 million.

For women across the globe, the pill was a landmark invention. For the first time in history, the choice of reproduction was placed in their hands.

In *Sexual Chemistry*, Lara V Marks publishes letters written to Dr Pincus by American women in the late 1950s. 'I am about 30 years old,' reads one. 'I have six children, the oldest little over seven, youngest a few days. My health don't (sic) seem to make from implanting even if it is fertilized. This relatively permanent contraceptive was immediately popular.

Women and HIV

By the early 1980s, women, especially in economically developed nations, were enjoying greater sexual freedom than ever before. Thanks to the wonders of modern antibiotics and the advent of the IUD,

---

it possible to go on this way. We have tried to be careful, but I get pregnant anyway. When I read about the pill , I couldn't help but cry, for I thought there is my ray of hope.'

While the pill has been a lifesaver for generations of women, early incarnations of the pill were linked to a number of health scares, including higher incidence of breast cancer, heart attacks and blood clots. Today, the newest pills are safer thanks largely to a reduction in the level of estrogen and progestin. Nevertheless, they provide no protection against sexually transmitted diseases. For two decades, this was often only a minor inconvenience. But in the early 1980s, an unexpected new infection redefined the meaning of safe sex. ◆

diaphragm and the pill, their sexual health was no longer at the mercy of men.

But today, HIV has again changed the rules of game. More than 75 per cent of HIV infections are transmitted through sex between men and women. Just over half of the 47 million currently HIV-positive people are female. Women are between two to four times more vulnerable to HIV than men, and they are being infected at a faster rate.

There are several biological reasons for women's increased susceptibility to HIV. During intercourse, more fluids are passed from men to women. Sperm also has a higher viral content than female sexual fluids. Another risk factor is that women have a greater area of mucous membrane exposed than men, and tears can also occur in vaginal (or rectal) tissue. The World Health Organization says this explains why young women, who are more likely to experience bleeding, may be especially susceptible to infection.

Indeed, many experts argue that HIV/AIDS is fast becoming a 'girls' epidemic'. WHO reports that young people (aged 15-24) account for half of all new HIV infections, and of these, two-thirds are female. In parts of sub-Saharan Africa, teenage girls are six times more likely to be infected than their male peers.

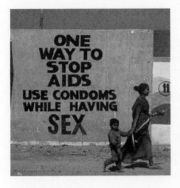

Certainly, the epidemic in Africa disproportionately affects women. Young women (15-24 years) in South Africa, for example, are four times more likely to be HIV-positive than young men: in 2005, 17 per cent of young women had HIV compared with 4.4 per cent in the male category. In Asia, infection rates have jumped 10 per cent among women in the last two years.

Beyond women's biological susceptibility and their inability to insist on contraception in many countries, there are additional social factors affecting infection rates. AIDS disproportionately affects the poorest, the most vulnerable and the least educated people in the world. Women often constitute the poorest of the poor, with low status and widespread illiteracy. They are vulnerable due to their weaker physique: many men just beat their partner if she refuses sex, or wants the man to wear a condom. Rape is common. This denial and lack of education places women at an ever-greater risk of infection than men.

Sex education

Lack of education is a fundamental driver in the spread of HIV. In Cambodia and Vietnam, surveys have shown that almost 50 per cent of young women aged 15-24 believe they can contract HIV from a mosquito bite, around 30 per cent by supernatural means, while nearly 35 per cent believe a healthy-looking person cannot be infected.

AIDS awareness is also very poor in China. One survey found at least 10 per cent of respondents in major cities did not know what the disease was; of those who did, a third thought it could be transmitted via toilet seats or towels. Another study on Chinese students aged 12-18 years found only 58 per cent knew two paths of transmission for HIV/AIDS.

The importance of educating women is even more significant given their role as mothers. In most Southern African countries, more than one in five pregnant women is HIV-positive. In Asia, HIV prevalence among pregnant women is much lower, but numbers are rising, and because of large population sizes, even an additional one per cent prevalence can mean hundreds of thousands of women.

With fewer than four per cent of couples in most developing countries relying on condoms, international development charities are calling for easier, inexpensive preventive products, such as such as microbicides and female condoms (see p 91). Were these introduced, they could have a huge impact. One recent study found that even if they were only used by 20 per cent of women already in contact with health services, some 2.5 million new HIV infections could be averted in three years.

The sex trade

Perhaps unsurprisingly, significantly higher rates of HIV infection than average have been documented among sex-workers and their clients. Female and young male sex-workers are unlikely to confront a rampant adult male with requests that he put on a condom. The sex industry is widely recognized as a common means of HIV infection entering the general population.

Female sex-workers are in the highest risk category in the fight against AIDS. Not only are they continually exposed to sexual intercourse, they are more likely to be drug users, and risk HIV-infection through unclean needles. Here too, lack of education presents a major barrier to safe sex. A WHO survey of sex-workers in Cambodia, for example, found 44 per cent had not been to school.

In some parts of the world, HIV rates among this group are rising. Nearly a quarter of female sex-workers in the Vietnamese capital, Ho Chi Minh City, are HIV-positive. In Guangxi province, China, prevalence among sex-workers rose to nearly 11 per cent in 2000 from 0 per cent in 1998.

Despite this bleak picture, according to UNAIDS, experiences in the field indicate that sex-workers are actually among those most likely to respond positively to HIV-prevention programs. Arguably the most successful example is the '100 per cent Condom Use Program' in Thailand and Cambodia. In the early 1990s, sex-workers were taught about sexual health and encouraged to insist on condoms. The results were astounding. Between 1989 and 1994, condom use rates in the sex industry rose from 14 per cent to 94 per cent in Thailand, with annual STI numbers falling from 400,000 to 30,000. WHO reports that condom use in Thailand and Cambodia has resulted in drops of HIV rates of more than 80 per cent since the peak of the epidemic. Today, commercial sex, which was once a major cause of HIV distribution, currently accounts for 'only' 21 per cent of infections in Cambodia and 16 per cent in Thailand.

This pro-condom approach has been repeated as far

afield as India and Brazil. International AIDS charity Avert reports that in the Kenyan capital of Nairobi, HIV prevention campaigns aimed at sex workers in the 1990s, including peer support and condom promotion, resulted in a reduction from 25-50 per cent to 4 per cent in HIV incidence amongst sex-workers in the city by the end of the decade.

The female condom

One of the most recent weapons in the fight against HIV has been a very different kind of condom altogether. Invented by a Danish physician in 1984, the female condom is a sheath worn inside the vagina, extending outward to cover the vulva. Globally, the female condom has many different brand names, including Reality, Femidom, Dominique, Femy, Myfemy, Protectiv' [sic] and Care. It is the only female contraceptive to provide effective protection against HIV.

Despite this cachet, the female condom has wholly failed to capture public imagination in Western countries. In 2005, the National Office of Statistics' report *Contraception and Sexual Behaviour* reported that UK usage is so low that it registers as 0 per cent. In the US, it is equally unpopular. This is due to negative perceptions

(British comedienne Jo Brand famously compared them to supermarket carrier bags) and the fact that Western women often have the economic and social power to insist on other forms of contraception.

Where HIV rates are highest, however, the female condom has proved a real success. In developing world countries, where women may be in no position to demand their men use condoms, having an effective choice of their own is invaluable.

While a 'rustling' sound during sex was a common complaint against the earliest female condoms, newer versions are much quieter. Nevertheless, these 'sound effects' can actually add to their attraction: in Senegal, for example, the female condom is sold with erotic beads, which are worn around the hips. When a woman moves, the beads make a similar sound to the condom. Senegalese women have also wryly suggested that the female condom is so large because their men are so well endowed.

In Asia, these condoms have also been marketed as a sexual enhancement. Sex education organization, the Pleasure Project, reports that sex-workers in Sri Lanka can charge more money for sex with the female condom than without it. According to their survey, more than 90 per cent of users claimed to enjoy the female condom, with nearly 60 per cent saying that their clients liked it and were excited to watch its insertion.

Today, approximately 14 million female condoms are distributed to women in the developing world every year. This compares to over 6,000 million male condoms. In November 2005, the World YWCA called on national health ministries and international donors to increase female condom provision by more than tenfold. They argued that female condoms remain the only tool for HIV prevention that women can initiate and control, but that 'they remain virtually inaccessible to women in the developing world due to their high cost of 72 cents per piece'. If 180 million female condoms were ordered, the price per unit would decline to approximately 22 cents.

Despite the differences in attitudes to condoms in all their shapes, sizes and manifestations, they have been a part of world culture – sniggered at, praised or vilified. The next chapter takes a look at condoms and the world of culture.

5 Plastic fantastic

'The condom is the glass slipper of our generation. You slip it on when you meet a stranger. You dance all night – then you throw it away. The condom, I mean. Not the stranger.'

CHUCK PALAHNIUK, US NOVELIST.

Throughout history, the humble condom has caught the public imagination in the most unexpected ways. From art galleries to hikers' backpacks, it has taken center stage in a variety of unlikely places. Along the way, it has earned a host of nicknames, taken on bizarre new shapes, colors and smells, and continues to evolve for every new generation.

The very first definitive account of a condom being used as a male contraceptive comes from 17th-century French literature. In the Parisian play, *L'Escole des Filles* [sic] penned in 1655, the character Susanne talks of 'use by the man of a small cloth' to prevent pregnancy. Writing half a century earlier, however, the English playwright William Shakespeare was already alluding to condoms. Never one to shy away from bawdy *double-entendres*, the Bard refers to the 'Venus glove' and 'quondam' – an early form of the word condom – in his tragedy *Troilus and Cressida*.

Condoms have captured other literary minds too. There are numerous references to 'rubber preservatives' in James Joyce's celebrated work, *Ulysses*, which was published in 1922. In the 1930s, authors George Orwell and Aldous Huxley also name-checked condoms in *Keep the Aspidistra Flying* and *Brave New World* respectively. British playwright and essayist George Bernard Shaw reportedly went even further, calling condoms 'the greatest invention of the 19th century'.

Use and abuse

While poets and playwrights have praised them in verse and prose, more practical thinkers have devised a variety of new uses for condoms.

The tough, waterproof nature of latex has found particular favor with the military. Earlier we saw how soldiers wrapped condoms around the muzzle of their rifles to stop dirt getting in. Indeed, in the first Gulf War, shares in Japan's largest condom manufacturer Okamotos Industries reportedly rose 10 per cent on the strength of market talk that US soldiers were fixing condoms onto their gun barrels to keep out sand. In battlefield hospitals,

URBAN MYTHS

In 1996, news began to spread about a mass of floating condoms spotted by scientists in the Pacific Ocean. This 'condom reef' reportedly measured up to two miles long, an eighth of a mile wide and in places up to 60 feet deep. The story was reported around the world, and still features on various news blogs and websites. It is entirely untrue. While no such reef ever appeared, there are however environmental concerns about the proper disposal of condoms. In 2003, for example, the US city of Milwaukee pledged $2 million to add a filtering system to a wastewater treatment plant to stop condoms floating out into Lake Michigan.

Another popular myth surrounding condoms is that wearing two condoms provides extra protection. This practice, known as 'double bagging', is often used by men going with prostitutes. Although intended to give the wearer twice the safety, double-bagging actually results in even greater danger, as there is a much higher risk of breakage due to the extra friction between the condoms. ◆

condoms have also doubled up as makeshift colostomy bags, while on long bomber trips, aircrew have also been known to pass urine into condoms and throw them over enemy territory.

On the ground, condoms are frequently used by hikers and campers to keep matches dry, and they are highly effective portable emergency water carriers. British SAS crews carry them for just this reason.

Criminals have also devised imaginative new uses for condoms. They are an especially popular vessel for drug smugglers, who stuff them with powder or tablets and either swallow them or insert them into the rectum.

On canvas

The very earliest pictorial description of a male sheath dates back to prehistoric times. There is the early cave painting at Les Combarelles mentioned in Chapter 1. It is impossible to know, however, whether the sheath depicted actually served any contraceptive purpose, or was simply decorative. One of the earliest conclusive examples of condoms on canvas is a self-portrait by the German artist Zoffany (1779). In this picture, the artist's own animal-gut prophylactics can be seen hanging underneath his mantelpiece.

In more recent times, condoms have also featured in the art world. Controversial British artist Tracey Emin's piece *My Bed*, which was short-listed for the 1999 Turner Prize, consisted of her own unmade bed, with sheets thrown back and used condoms and menstrual blood-stained underwear clearly on view.

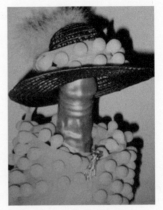

One of Renate Bertlmann's extraordinary images.

Self-styled 'anti-pornographic' artist Renate Bertlmann frequently uses condoms in her gallery installations. In *Präservativwurfmesser* ('Condom throwing knife'), she creates a catapult in the form of two penis shafts, and a cartridge belt decorated with stuffed condoms. In *Fleurs du Mal*, she arranges textured condoms into colorful artificial flowers.

Brazilian artist Adriana Bertini also celebrates condoms through her art. Many of her paintings, sculptures, picture frames and brightly colored women's dresses are made from factory-reject condoms. Her creations are intended to raise awareness and inspire reflection about condom use, and foster discussion about the global HIV/AIDS crisis.

Condoms at the cinema

Given the US movie industry's obsession with sexual relationships, HIV/AIDS campaigners argue that it is ideally placed to emphasize the important of safe sex. In reality, however, contraception very rarely appears on-screen. In 2004, a team of doctors accused Hollywood of irresponsibility over its portrayal of sex after its review of some of the biggest blockbusters from the last 20 years showed that only one movie made reference to a condom.

Writing in the journal of the Royal Society of Medicine, Dr Gunasekera and his co-authors Simon Chapman and Sharon Campbell reported that none of the top 200 films promoted safe sex, while nobody ended up with an unwanted pregnancy or any infection.

They noted that in 98 per cent of sexual episodes, which could have resulted in pregnancy, no form of birth control was used or even suggested. Particular offenders included *Basic Instinct* (1992), *American Pie* (2001) and the Bond film *Die Another Day* (2002). In *American Pie*, which has seven sex scenes, all involving new partners with no condoms or birth control measures, the only

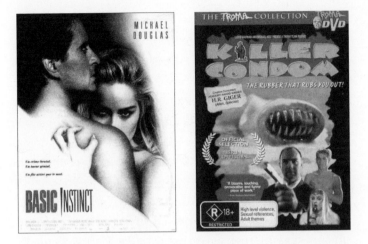

consequence of condom use was 'social embarrassment'.

Only one film has put condoms truly center stage, albeit not especially helpfully. *Killer Condom* (originally *Kondom des Grauens*) is a 1997 shock-horror comedy movie, based on a comic book by German cartoonist Ralf Koenig. The story focuses on a college professor, who has a nasty encounter with a condom when trying to seduce an attractive female student. The prophylactic in question has somehow grown razor-sharp teeth and developed a thirst for blood. When it bites off the professor's manhood, a team of detectives is assigned to hunt down this new breed of killer condoms.

Let's get it on

More songs are written about love than anything else. From Marvin Gaye to Metallica, artists of every color, creed and genre have embraced love – and lovemaking – through their music. Despite this age-old tradition of sonic seduction, however, safe sex almost never gets a mention. The most obvious reason is that while condoms are functional and practical, they are rarely considered to be 'sexy'.

While most music-makers simply ignore condoms, some genres have been accused of actively promoting unsafe sex. In their overtly sexualized music videos, many US rap artists reduce women to ass-shaking sexual objects, while they act out fantasies of being the 'pimp'. It is noticeable that condoms are almost always entirely absent. And studies have shown that this may affect the sexual behavior of the viewers. In 2003, a comparative survey was made between women who had regular exposure to rap music videos and those who did not. In the *American Journal of Public Health*, the authors revealed that the first group of women was 110 per cent more likely to 'never use condoms'.

In 2006, fellow US rapper Ludacris, known for his explicit lyrics about sex, drugs and violence, began to

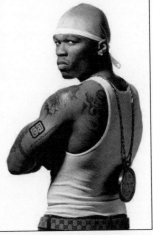
speak out about safe sex. 'I talk a lot about sex in my music, but you don't ever hear me talk about condoms,' he told students in Chicago. 'I can't speak for other rappers, but I think it's important that I let you know to be safe when you're having sex. Young people need to know about HIV/AIDS before it is too late, so it's extremely important that we talk about it.'

Afrobeat musician Femi Kuti, the son of legendary Nigerian musician Fela Kuti, has long been committed to spreading the safe-sex message. After signing up to an AIDS campaign, Kuti commented in a UNICEF report in 2000 that 'failing to educate people about the disease is like signing their death sentence'. Kuti has even taken the pro-condom message into songs such as 'Stop AIDS':

If you must do sha!

You better cover your bamboo.

Remmy Ongala, born in DR Congo, is another musician committed to communicating a safe-sex message. In 1990, he released a song called 'Mambo Kwa Socks' (Things With Socks), a reference to Tanzanian slang for condoms. The song was a plea to young African men to help slow the spread of AIDS by practicing safe sex.

Thanks to Dr Grigoriy Chausovskiy, there is now an even closer connection between condoms and music. The Ukrainian scientist has invented the world's first musical condom. The rubber, which works like a normal

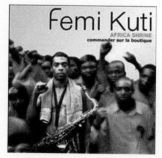

contraceptive, has tiny sensors connected to a miniature electronic drive. Nevertheless, the doctor says there is no danger of being electrocuted. According to the instructions, the music gets louder as the sex gets more vigorous, while different lovemaking positions determine what tune is played.

Novelty acts

Modern condoms come in all shapes and sizes. They are also available in almost every conceivable color. While most are either transparent or pink, in *Johnny Come Lately*, Jeannette Parisot reports that Kenyans especially like red condoms, the Japanese prefer black and baby blue, and in Egypt, Thailand, Jamaica and other warm climes, blues, greens, pinks and yellows are most popular.

To spice up oral sex, there is a variety of flavored

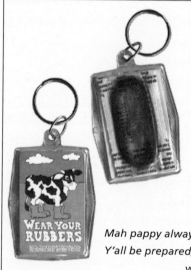

'Battered condoms like those carried around in wallets and purses may fail when used. Protect yourself and your lover with one of these cool key chain designs – makes a great gift, too!

High impact clear polystyrene for durability. Easily opened with a coin.'

Mah pappy always said, 'Son, be prepared.' Y'all be prepared, too, all right?

www.condom.com/kp.html

condoms. Popular ones include strawberry, vanilla, banana, apple, coconut, spearmint, chocolate, orange and kiwi fruit. For tougher taste buds, there are prophylactics on sale flavored with tequila or curry.

Thanks to advances in latex technology, condoms can now be made to look like pretty much anything. But outlandish creations, such as condoms with elephant heads or ones which glow in the dark, are intended to be for foreplay only, and are not safe to be worn as contraceptives. They often have holes or risk falling apart and causing internal damage.

People wanting even more protection than regular-shaped condoms do have another alternative, however. The 'anti-VD sheath' covers both the wearer's penis and testicles, thereby preventing an even larger part of the

STICK IT ON

In December 2006, researchers at the German Institute for Condom Consultancy announced plans to launch a spray-on condom. According to reports, the institute will develop a spray can into which the man inserts his penis, which is then sprayed with latex from nozzles on all sides. The aim is to create an effective contraceptive that fits better than a standard condom and hence does not slip.

In China, meanwhile, scientists have already experimented with liquid condoms. In 2005, the *China Daily* newspaper reported the successful launch of the country's first 'condom-in-a-can'. An antiseptic foam, which is sprayed onto the penis, it reportedly 'forms a physical membrane inside the vagina, protecting it from infection, acting as a barrier to pregnancy and providing a lubricating effect.' ◆

anatomy coming into contact with the sexual partner.

Condoms are also being used as a way to combat sexual violence. In South Africa, a new anti-rape female condom has been successfully trialed and will soon be on sale. Lined with 25 razor-sharp teeth, the Rapex condom fastens onto an attacker's penis if he attempts penetration.

6 In our hands

Five centuries after Fallopio's first linen sheaths and several millennia after people began experimenting with contraception, the condom has become a truly global icon. The single most effective weapon in the fight against HIV/AIDS, this cheap strip of latex is arguably more important now than ever before.

Nevertheless, our historically complex relationship with the condom continues to be shaped by a variety of factors, from economic might and political will to cultural and religious beliefs. As we journey into the 21st century, there are still many lessons to learn, and hurdles yet to overcome.

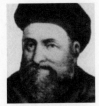

Gabriele Fallopio

Supply and demand

The global condom market is worth several billion dollars. Between six and nine billion male condoms are currently distributed by the global public sector each year, with an additional three to four billion units sold through commercial channels. The condom industry

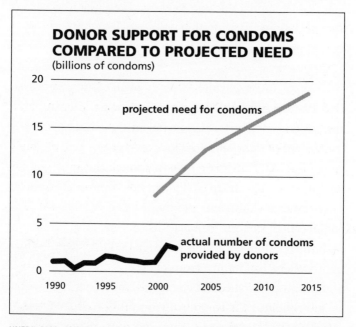

DONOR SUPPORT FOR CONDOMS COMPARED TO PROJECTED NEED
(billions of condoms)

projected need for condoms

actual number of condoms provided by donors

UNFPA, 2002. *Global Estimates of Contraceptive Commodities and Condoms for STI/HIV Prevention, 2000-2015*. New York: UNFPA. UNFPA, 2004. *Database on Donor Support for Contraceptives and Logistics Management*. New York: UNFPA.

is forecasted to grow, especially in Asia and Central Africa. There will also be greater product differentiation in terms of shapes, sizes and more advanced flavors, alongside other new developments in male contraception (see p 117).

Nevertheless, it is clear that condom supply needs to rise fast to combat the world's HIV/AIDS epidemic. Across the developing world in particular, condom provision currently falls well short of demand.

Greater condom provision would have a great impact in poor countries, which already struggle to effectively deliver the safe sex message. According to campaign group Make Poverty History, young people who have completed primary education are less than half as likely to contract HIV as those missing an education. It argues that universal primary education would prevent 700,000 cases of HIV-infection, almost 30 per cent of all new infections in this age group.

Poverty is closely tied to lack of education. While Western economies prospered in the nine years between 1995 and 2004, the number of people living in poverty in sub-Saharan Africa grew by 140 million. International NGO Social Watch says that 'extreme poverty is not declining and actually increasing in Africa, Latin America, the Middle East, Eastern Europe and most of Asia, where progress is concentrated in China, India and Vietnam.'

This poverty affects HIV prevalence in numerous ways. Besides having fewer education opportunities, a person with HIV will almost certainly be unable to afford the anti-retroviral drugs (ARVs) necessary to keep the disease at bay for a number of years.

While advances in science and better health campaigns saw the number of AIDS deaths fall in the US in 1997, this pattern was not repeated in poorer parts of the world. One year of ARV therapy costs in the region of $15,000. For the one billion-plus people living on less than a dollar a day, such vital, life-prolonging treatment is out of reach.

Plans to make cheaper generic drugs have been welcomed by charities and NGOs. But even they are likely to cost approximately $400 per person per year. In Africa, according to British charity Christian Aid, the average spend per person on health is currently just $10 and as low as $3 in some countries.

Besides an absence of financial resources, and proper HIV education, many countries have shown little political will to address the problem. One reason is the disease's 'gay' connotations. In many homophobic societies in the developing world, AIDS has historically been considered a gay disease; its existence was therefore often simply denied. In fact, more than 80 per cent of HIV transmission in Africa is now heterosexual.

Condom fatigue

Low condom use is not always linked to availability. Even in those countries where condoms *are* widely available, unsafe sex is frequently practiced. Britain currently has the highest teenage pregnancy rates in Europe. In surveys, almost a third of 15-year-olds admitted to not using a condom the last time they had sex. In the last 10 years, the number of chlamydia (a sexually transmitted infection) cases in the UK has risen almost 250 per cent for girls and 500 per cent for boys. The reasons for this trend include lack of sex education and ignorance (or underestimation) of the dangers of unprotected sex. Among older age groups, however, there are often no such excuses. Here, the decline in condom use is frequently ascribed to boredom with the safe sex message.

This is not the first instance of so-called 'condom fatigue'. Those born in the post-war 'baby boom' period developed their sexual behavior well before the outbreak of HIV/AIDS redefined the importance of contraception. For many, those liberal attitudes continue to shape their

BAREBACKING

The riskiest form of sex for transmitting HIV is unprotected anal intercourse (UAI). Among gay men, the practice is known as 'barebacking'. No one knows the exact scale of unprotected gay sex globally, but it is recognized as a significant contributor in the spread of HIV/AIDS.

Unlike for many people in the developing world, for example, one unique characteristic of UAI in wealthier nations is that its practitioners often understand the risks, have access to condoms, and yet still refuse to wear them.

In 1990, almost a decade after the outbreak of the virus, a survey of gay men in San Francisco showed that 18 per cent had engaged in UAI in the past year. In 1991, an AIDS Action Committee of Massachusetts survey revealed that one in three gay men questioned admitted to having anal intercourse without a condom.

US psychologist Ron Stall suggests that this prevalence of sexual risk-taking in the gay community can be a result of 'a variety of psychosocial health issues, including depression, anti-gay violence, childhood sexual abuse, and substance abuse'. Additional factors may include negative attitudes towards condom use, internalized homophobia and a sense of

sex lives. Post-menopausal women and older men also appear more likely to take risks. In 2006, a study by the American Association of Retired Persons (AARP) found inevitability of becoming infected with HIV.

There have also been even more sinister reasons. Filled with a sense of their own doom, some HIV-positive men deliberately infect other people through unprotected sex. In 2007, a 48-year-old married Melbourne man went on trial for knowingly spreading HIV to other men. He allegedly bragged that he had made '75 people pos' and regularly held 'conversion parties' to create more people with HIV so that he could have bareback sex – the 'logic' here being that if they all are HIV-positive it does not matter if they have unprotected sex.

For a very small minority of uninfected barebackers, this practice has even eroticized HIV. The slang 'bug chaser' is often used to describe non-infected gay men who deliberately seek to become infected with HIV.

A far greater number of younger gay barebackers however are simply unaware or in denial about HIV risk altogether, having grown up in an era of more advanced anti-retroviral drugs (ARVs).

Nevertheless, the implications of barebacking remain as lethal as ever. New York historian Charles Kaiser argues that 'a person who is HIV-positive has no more right to unprotected intercourse than he has to put a bullet through another person's head'. ◆

that 76 per cent of single Americans aged 45 and over don't use protection when having sex.

'It's because the over-50 crowd doesn't use condoms,'

Dr Margaret New told NBC. 'They can't get pregnant. They haven't been brought up with that fear that they had to use condoms.' As a result, the rate of sexually transmitted disease among baby-boomers is growing at an alarming rate. According to the US Centers for Disease Control and Prevention (CDC), AIDS cases among people age 50 and older in the US jumped 22 per cent between 1991 and 2004.

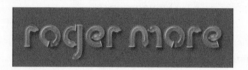

Britain's advertising watchdog has ruled that a billboard poster for a brand of condoms should be removed because it was likely to cause 'serious or widespread offence'. The Advertising Standards Authority said it had received four complaints about the poster for Durex's Performa Condoms.

The ad featured a number of condoms inflated to create the words 'roger more'. Durex's parent company, SSL International, defended the advert, saying the term 'to roger' was an 'antiquated and comic reference to sex'. They said the poster was 'intended to promote safe sex and enjoyment'. 'We believe that promoting greater use of condoms is also a socially responsible activity,' said John Flaherty of Durex. ◆

BBC, 21 May 2003.

In wealthy nations, medical advances have also contributed to a more laissez-faire attitude to condom use. As treatments for people with HIV/AIDS have improved, so fear of contracting HIV has fallen. As a result, unprotected sex can increasingly appear less dangerous. In 2004, Britain's National Institute for Health and Clinical Excellence (NICE) reported that the 21st century 'heralds a trend towards more sexual risk-taking throughout Europe, with sharp increases in the rates of sexually transmitted infections'.

New face of male contraception

For centuries, the condom has been the only reliable artificial form of male contraception. Despite changes to its material and design, the basic concept has never changed. Besides *coitus interruptus*, a man's only other recourse to safe sex has been more drastic. Vasectomy, also known as male sterilization, is a small out-patient operation that stops sperm from the testes being ejaculated during intercourse. Although a permanent method of birth control, and much cheaper to perform that female sterilization, it can often be reversed. However, it offers no protection against HIV or other sexually transmitted diseases.

Looking to the future, there are a plethora of new alternative male contraceptive treatments in development. Adjudin is a drug that disrupts the process of sperm maturation in the testes for a limited period of time. As yet untested on humans, it has been successfully trialed in rats. Scientists are currently working on a gel or implant version for male use.

The 'dry orgasm' pill is another product in the pipeline. Men using this pill would experience an orgasm that feels normal, but produce a decreased volume of semen containing little to no sperm. The drug would take effect within 2-3 hours of ingestion, and wear off within 24 hours. A man could take this pill as needed before having sex.

For many years, plans for a male version of the female oral contraceptive pill hinged on gossypol. Derived from a cotton plant, this chemical has strong contraceptive properties, and formed the base of several trials carried out in the 1980s and 1990s. The drug proved too effective however – causing extremely high rates of permanent infertility. In 1998, the World Health Organization's Research Group on Methods for the Regulation of Male Fertility recommended that gossypol research should be abandoned. But it could have a role for men who have completed their families.

JACOB ZUMA SPOKESPERSON FOR CONDOM COMPANY?

It's well known that South Africans are ingenious when it comes to left-field inventiveness – think Kreepy Krawly, the CAT scan and the wind-up radio – but this raises the bar, so to speak. A Cape Town based inventor has created a quick-draw condom to 'keep the momentum going', and who better to be the spokesperson than Zuma? (The South African former vice-president who was charged with attempted rape; he was subsequently cleared.) ◆

Posted in *Real Life Stories* by Fred on 25 October 2006.

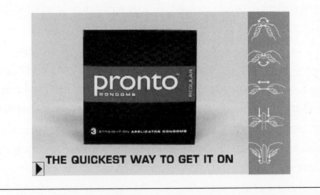

Recent improvements have also been made to the latex condom. After researching South Africa's AIDS problem, condom designer Willem van Rensburg found that many people don't wear condoms because they are considered

NUMBER-CRUNCHING

Condoms have also been cited in the fight against global warming. In May 2007, the UK environmental think-tank Optimum Population Trust (OPT) claimed that having a large family should be regarded as an eco-crime. A lower birth rate, it argued, would help to slash national carbon dioxide emissions. With each UK citizen creating nearly 750 tonnes of carbon dioxide in a lifetime, the OPT estimated a 'climate cost' of each Briton equivalent to roughly £30,000. As a result, the cost of a projected 10 million increase in the UK population by 2074 would be more than £300 billion. *The Guardian* noted that a condom for 35p therefore represented a 'spectacular' potential return. ◆

unsexy. 'People find it's a passion-killer and they're willing to take their chances,' he told the BBC in 2006. Van Rensburg's Pronto condoms, which do not need to be unwrapped, are designed not to spoil the moment. Thanks to a special plastic applicator inside the condom packet, they take just one second to put on.

Positive trends

In 2004, the UN's Department of Economic and Social Affairs reported that the majority (61 per cent) of the world's couples of reproductive age regularly use contraception, including condoms.

According to the report:

♦ 69 per cent of couples in 'developed' countries use contraception.

♦ 59 per cent of couples in 'less developed' countries use contraception.

♦ Contraceptive use has increased by at least one percentage point per year in 56 per cent of all developing countries.

♦ In Africa, the percentage of contraceptive users increased from 17 per cent in 1990 to 28 per cent in 2000.

♦ In Asia, it increased from 57 per cent to 65 per cent.

♦ In Latin America and the Caribbean, it rose from 62 per cent to 74 per cent.

Call to arms

Parental choice. Peace of mind. Protection. We use condoms for very different purposes – at different times in our lives. And yet there remains one common factor in our colorful relationship with the sheath: male domination. Even today, half a millennium after their first modern incarnation, men are still most likely to decide on whether condoms are used or not.

But this greater say must also bring extra responsibility. Today more than ever, men should feel duty-bound

CONDOMS AND RAINFORESTS

A new condom factory in Brazil is aiming to meet the country's contraception shortfall and ease rainforest destruction at the same time. 'Brazilians need to use 1.2 billion condoms a year to prevent the spread of AIDS,' Alessandro Grangeiro, Brazil's AIDS program co-ordinator, told BBC World Service's *Science in Action* program: 'The Government is distributing today 700 million. So the factory will make the whole situation a lot better.'

The factory, in Xapuri, a remote province in the northwestern state of Acre, will bring cheaper condoms and sustainable development to the region. It also hopes to reduce the pressure on land clearance in the region. 'You won't have to destroy (rubber trees) anymore,' said Jose Maria Barbossa Bakierno, of the National Rubber-Tappers' Council. 'Now, we can make a profit by preserving them. The hope is that the development of the latex industry to make condoms will increase the market for rubber, and mean the trees will not have to be cut down to make land for farming.' ◆

to practice safe sex and protect their partners from unnecessary health risks. After all, not only can their sexual behavior directly help thwart the devastating spread of HIV/AIDS, it can also prevent unwanted pregnancies and painful, often life-threatening abortions. This is true sexual power – the ability to stop unnecessary disease and death, and create life only when intended by both parties.

In the age of HIV/AIDS, condoms have given us the best of both worlds. Thanks to them, and despite counter-claims by conservative religious groups, safe sex does not demand total abstinence. And unlike female

FCUK-ING JUST DO IT!

Imagine if major companies from all around the world started producing or sponsoring condoms. They would become fashionable and companies would probably advertise more openly. Just a few examples...

◆ Nike Condoms – Just do it.
◆ Peugeot Condoms – The ride of your life.
◆ KFC Condoms – Finger Licking Good.
◆ Burger King Condoms – Home of the Whopper.
◆ M&Ms Condoms – Melt in your mouth, not in your hands.
◆ Coca-Cola Condoms – The Real Thing.
◆ Ever Ready Condoms – Keep going and going...
◆ Goodyear Condoms – For a longer ride go wide.
◆ Nokia condoms – Connecting people.
◆ One-2-One condoms – Who would you most like to have a 1-2-1 with?
◆ Windows condoms – Plug and Play.
◆ FCUK condoms – No comment required!

contraceptives, which often come with side-effects (the pill) or discomfort (IUDs), the male condom is a simple, non-invasive, cheap and incredibly effective tool.

So it is time we celebrated the condom as a true global success story. Of course, not everywhere is its potential yet fully recognized. When one sexual health worker visited a remote farming community in central Ethiopia, he reportedly demonstrated how to put on a condom by unrolling it onto his fingers. On his return to the same village nine months later, he was accosted by an angry farmer. The man said he had put the condom on his fingers during sex as instructed, but still his wife fell pregnant.

Contacts

ACT UP (AIDS Coalition to Unleash Power)
www.actupny.org

Avert – international AIDS charity
www.avert.org

The AIDS Support Organization (Uganda)
www.taso.co.ug

The Global Fund to Fight AIDS, TB and Malaria
www.globalfund.org

The Global Network of People Living with HIV//AIDS (GNP+)
www.gnpplus.net

Marie Stopes International
www.mariestopes.org

Médecins Sans Frontières
www.msf.org

Netdoctor contraceptive advice
www.netdoctor.co.uk

Oxfam
www.oxfam.org

The Site contraceptive advice
www.thesite.org

Treatment Action Campaign (South Africa)
www.tac.org.za

UNAIDS - The Joint United Nations Programme on HIV/AIDS
www.unaids.org

UNFPA - UN Population Fund
www.unfpa.org

WHO –World Health Organization
www.who.int

TRIGGER ISSUES FROM NEW INTERNATIONALIST

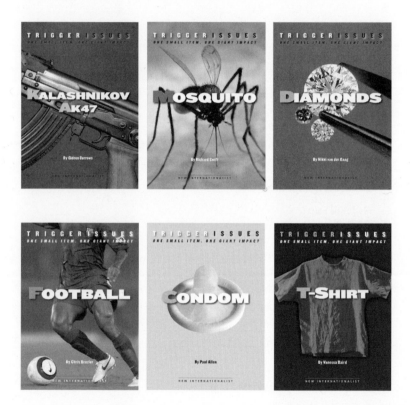

ABOUT THE NEW INTERNATIONALIST

The New Internationalist is an independent not-for-profit publishing co-operative. Our mission is to report on issues of world poverty and inequality; to focus attention on the unjust relationship between the powerful and the powerless worldwide; to debate and campaign for the radical changes necessary if the needs of all are to be met.

We publish informative, timely current affairs titles and popular reference complemented by world food, photography and alternative gift books as well as calendars and diaries, maps and posters – all with a global justice world view.

We also publish the monthly *New Internationalist* magazine. Each month tackles a different subject such as the Oceans, Iran, Ethical Shopping or Darfur.

For more information, online ordering and trade order details: **www.newint.org**